Contemporary Diagnosis and Management of
Multiple Sclerosis®

Richard A. Rudick, MD

Director, Mellen Center for Multiple
Sclerosis Treatment and Research
Hazel Prior Hostetler Professor
of Neurology
Chairman, Division of Clinical Research
Cleveland Clinic Foundation
Cleveland, Ohio

D1636063

First Edi

Published by
Handbooks in Health Care Co.,
Newtown, Pennsylvania, USA

This book has been prepared and is presented as a service to the medical community. The information provided reflects the knowledge, experience, and personal opinions of the author, Richard A. Rudick, MD, Director, Mellen Center for Multiple Sclerosis Treatment and Research, and the Hazel Prior Hostetler Professor of Neurology, and Chairman, Division of Clinical Research, Cleveland Clinic Foundation, Cleveland, Ohio.

Acknowledgments
Dr. Rudick would like to acknowledge Karen Nichols, MEd, CHES, for her outstanding assistance in preparing this handbook and Bruce Trapp, PhD, for providing figures 5-6 and 5-7.

This book is not intended to replace or to be used as a substitute for the complete prescribing information prepared by each manufacturer for each drug. Because of possible variations in drug indications, in dosage information, in newly described toxicities, in drug/drug interactions, and in other items of importance, reference to such complete prescribing information is definitely recommended before any of the drugs discussed are used or prescribed.

International Standard Book Number: 1-931981-33-7

Library of Congress Catalog Card Number: 2004107350

Table of Contents

3

Chapter 1

Definition, History, and Epidemiology of Multiple Sclerosis

Multiple sclerosis (MS) is an inflammatory disease of the central nervous system (CNS) that damages myelin and CNS axons. It is generally categorized as an organ-specific autoimmune disease. It affects women more frequently than men (ratio of 3:2), most commonly begins around age 30, and is characterized in the early stages by episodic relapses and remissions. Table 1-1 lists the essential clinical features of MS. In its later stages, progressive neurologic impairment and disability occur. Multiple sclerosis is the most common disabling neurologic disease of young adults.

History of Multiple Sclerosis

The earliest account of a disease likely to have been MS comes from 14th century writings describing the illness of a Dutch nun, who fell ill at age 15. Within a few years, she developed difficulty walking, leg numbness, and intermittent blindness in one eye. She later developed difficulty swallowing and died 4 days short of her 53rd birthday. Augustus d'Este provided a more detailed description of possible MS in 1822. Ten months after his first transient symptoms, he developed transient double vision, and later leg weakness. He had repeated relapses with remission, but gradually increasing disability led to his death 26 years later.

**Table 1-1: Essential Clinical Features
of Multiple Sclerosis**

- Peak age range of onset is 18 to 35 years.

- Approximately 2/3 of patients are female.

- The disease follows a relapsing-remitting
  course at onset in 85% of cases, but is
  progressive from onset in 15%.

- 85% of relapsing cases eventually enter a
  secondary progressive phase.

- A progressive course from onset is more
  common in older-onset patients (>40 years).

- Multifocal pathology causes variable
  combinations of visual, motor, sensory,
  and cognitive manifestations.

Charcot is credited with the first comprehensive account of the features of MS, published in 1868. In a remarkable series of lectures, he characterized pathologic and clinical features of MS ('The nerve tubes...have become still more slender. Many of them have disappeared; in reality, they have been merely deprived of their medullary sheaths, and are now only represented by their axis-cylinders....') and demonstrated demyelination through his pathologic studies. The concept of MS as a disease primarily affecting myelin, with relative sparing of the neuronal elements, has persisted for more than 100 years. Evidence for widespread axonal injury has recently emerged, however, and it is now clear that the pathologic process in MS targets both myelin and axons. Charcot described perivascular inflammatory cuffs and macrophages in the actively demyelinating lesions. Thus, Charcot initially described MS as an inflammatory demyelinating disease, a fundamental concept about pathogenesis that persists to the present. Charcot described relapses and remissions, intention tremor, optic neuritis, and cerebral, spinal, and mixed forms of the disease. He even described less-common features of MS, such as bipolar symptoms and pathologic laughing and weeping.

Among Charcot's more remarkable conclusions was that demyelinated fibers can conduct the nerve impulse. Optic neuritis, he said, '...very rarely issues in complete blindness. This is peculiarly worthy of notice, especially if you remember that patches of sclerosis have been found, after death, occupying the whole thickness of the nerve trunks in the optic nerves, in cases, where during life, an enfeeblement of sight simply had been found. This apparent disproportion between the symptom and the lesion constitutes one of the most powerful arguments which can be invoked to show that the functional continuity of the nerve tubes is not absolutely interrupted...'. This statement long antedates more recent detailed observations confirming his observation and describing the physiology of conduction in demyelinated fibers.

An important development in our understanding of MS dates to the early 1930s, when experimental autoimmune encephalomyelitis (EAE) was developed as an experimental animal model for the disease. Much of modern scientific understanding of cell-mediated autoimmunity stems from studies of EAE. Understanding of MS has advanced rapidly with new developments such as electron microscopy; single fiber electrophysiologic techniques; patch clamp recording from single ion channels; evoked potentials; new histologic methods; cell culture techniques; new methods in molecular virology and immunology; magnetic resonance imaging and spectroscopy; and increasingly sophisticated clinical trial methodology. Despite these advances, Charcot's initial clinical descriptions of more than 100 years ago remain remarkably accurate and comprehensive.

Epidemiology

Multiple sclerosis is among the most common acquired neurologic diseases of young adults in the temperate zones. It accounts for more disability, more cost in care, and more lost income than any other neurologic disease in this age group in Western Europe and North America. Epidemiologic studies have demonstrated that MS has an unequal geographic distribution, with significant regional variations and variability within regions. Case-control studies have failed to identify consistent environmental factors that contribute to MS risk, and the relative contribution of genetic vs environmental factors is hotly debated.

Geographic Distribution

There is a distinct north-south gradient in the distribution of MS. The disease is rare in the tropics and increases in frequency at higher latitudes north, and probably also south, of the equator. The prevalence in the United States is reported at 57.8 per 100,000 but increases in a continuous fashion with increasing latitude. Below the 37th parallel, the prevalence is reported at 35.5, and above it at 68 per 100,000. A similar north-south gradient exists in Western Europe. The relationship between MS and latitude has been questioned in Europe, but is said to be present and unrelated to ancestral background in Australia and New Zealand, where the disease appears to increase with latitude south. A north-south gradient has not been demonstrated in Japan or Asia, where the prevalence is much lower. The incidence (number of new cases per 100,000 population per year) is said to be increasing in Olmsted County, Minnesota, but not in Iceland. The prevalence rate (number of cases per 100,000 population) has been increasing, probably because of better recognition of MS and improved treatment of complications with a correspondingly increased longevity of those affected.

Within the latitudinal gradient, certain regions have particularly high prevalence rates. In a 1956 survey by Sutherland, the overall prevalence in Scotland was 60 per

100,000. The Orkney Islands, north of Scotland, had a prevalence of 309 per 100,000 in 1980. In Norway, prevalence rates are consistently higher inland than they are along the coast. The prevalence in France was also found to differ significantly by region. A significant clustering of MS cases occurred in the northeastern part of France, and a significantly lower-prevalence area appeared in the south and west. These differences in geographic region, and the variability within regions, have raised a tantalizing suggestion of environmental factors, but so far no extrinsic environmental factor has been linked to the disease.

Migration Studies

Migration studies suggest that the risk of acquiring MS is established around the time of puberty. The most extensive and reliable studies of migrant populations were conducted among US military service veterans by John Kurtzke. Using location of birth and place of entry into active service as evidence of migration, he found that individuals migrating from high- to low-risk areas had a decrease in their expected risk of developing MS. Conversely, migration from low- to high-risk areas resulted in an increased risk of acquiring MS. Age at migration suggested that the risk of acquiring the disease in high-risk areas is established by about 15 years of age. Data on migration from low-risk to high-risk areas are less reliable, but the evidence suggests there is some increase in risk even in those older than 15 years of age at migration.

Clusters

MS clusters have been reported. Campbell reported one of the most famous, in which MS developed in 4 of 7 scientists who had studied swayback in sheep. These cases began within a few months of each other and within a few years of the scientists' common exposure. Many methodologic issues complicate interpretation of clusters, however. A reported cluster of MS in Galion, Ohio, illustrates some of the difficulties. The prevalence of MS in this small town was found to be high—112 cases per 100,000 in

June 1987. On closer inspection, though, it was suggested that the prevalence may have been artificially high because the population of the town had steadily decreased as the manufacturing base declined in the 1970s. Clinicians speculated that the residents of Galion who had MS remained in town, while the disease-free population migrated from the area, leaving an apparently high prevalence of MS. A case-control study failed to demonstrate occupational or industrial exposure or other environmental factors that could explain an increased risk of MS. Finally, it was difficult to know whether the prevalence in this town was actually higher than expected, because the expected prevalence is usually only a gross estimate from large geographic surveys in the region of interest.

Exposures

A reported cluster in a factory in Rochester, NY, is particularly interesting. The plant used elemental and ionic zinc to build parts for the automobile industry. Stein and coworkers reported 11 cases of clinically definite MS in a total employee population of 5,039, representing a calculated incidence of 21.8 per 100,000 per year. Even after age adjustment, this figure is far higher than that reported in the areas of highest-known MS incidence. The cluster was interesting because the erythrocytes of MS patients were reported to be high in membrane-bound zinc. Tests of serum zinc in MS patients and other employees showed some elevation over out-of-plant controls, but no definite conclusions about the role of zinc in MS could be drawn. A case-control study prompted by the Stein report failed to confirm increased MS cases or an association with zinc levels in a different, similar automotive plant.

Cook and associates presented evidence for elevated levels of antibodies to canine distemper virus in MS patients, and raised the possibility that MS might be caused by human infection with distemper virus, transmitted by exposure to dogs. There is no consensus on the relationship between canine distemper virus and MS at present.

Epidemics

Some evidence indicates that environmental factors other than latitude may be important in explaining the geographic pattern of MS. Reports of point-source epidemics are the most interesting. An epidemic of MS was reported in the Faeroe Islands, located northwest of the Orkney Islands. Because of their geographic location and ethnic makeup, the Faeroe Islands would be expected to have a high prevalence of MS. However, MS appears to have been rare before 1940, and to have sharply increased after World War II. Kurtzke and colleagues reported no evidence for the disease before 1943. Between 1943 and 1960, 24 cases appeared, but after 1960, only one case developed. Kurtzke also reported evidence that an epidemic occurred in Iceland at about the same time. The situation in Iceland was less clear because of a higher background frequency of the disease. Kurtzke argued that these studies strongly supported environmental factors that resulted in a high MS incidence, beginning in the early 1940s. One possibility was the movement of British and American troops into these areas during World War II, but the exact nature of the introduced environmental factor remains to be elucidated. Kurtzke has further reported that beginning in 1943 and every 13 years thereafter, four successive MS epidemics occurred in the Faeroes (clinical MS was then thought to arise as the late sequelae of the primary exposure). He concluded that the evidence supports the presence of a transmissible agent, with the period at risk for acquiring MS occurring between the ages of 13 and 26. He further speculated that the transmissible agent is a virus that widely infects the target population, but only rarely results in clinical MS. The suggestion of a transmissible agent remains controversial but interesting.

The epidemiologic and migration studies support the possibility that environmental exposure occurs in childhood, most likely around the time of puberty, influencing an individual's susceptibility to MS. The epidemiologic studies have identified a number of putative toxins and infectious agents, but none has been proven relevant. Recent genetic studies strongly suggest that the disease is polygenic, and further suggest that genetic factors may be as important—or even more important than—environmental factors.

Suggested Readings

Compston A: The 150th anniversary of the first depiction of the lesions of multiple sclerosis. *J Neurol Neurosurg Psychiatry* 1988;51:1249-1252.

Cook SD: Multiple sclerosis and viruses. *Mult Scler* 1997;3:388-389.

Dean G: Was there an epidemic of multiple sclerosis in the Faeroe Islands? *Neuroepidemiology* 1988;7:165-167.

Fredrikson S, Kam-Hansen S: The 150-year anniversary of multiple sclerosis: does its early history give an etiological clue? *Perspect Biol Med* 1989;32:237-243.

Gilden DH: A search for virus in multiple sclerosis. *Hybrid Hybridomics* 2002;21:93-97.

Hickey WF: The pathology of multiple sclerosis: a historical perspective. *J Neuroimmunol* 1999;98:37-44.

Kurtzke JF, Hyllested K: Multiple sclerosis in the Faeroe Islands: I. Clinical and epidemiological features. *Ann Neurol* 1979;5:6-21.

Kurtzke JF, Hyllested K: Multiple sclerosis in the Faeroe Islands. II. Clinical update, transmission, and the nature of MS. *Neurology* 1986;36:307-328.

McDonald WI: The dynamics of multiple sclerosis. The Charcot Lecture. *J Neurol* 1993;240:28-36.

McDonnell GV, Hawkins SA: Multiple sclerosis in Northern Ireland: a historical and global perspective. *Ulster Med J* 2000;69:97-105.

Poser CM: Viking voyages: the origin of multiple sclerosis? An essay in medical history. *Acta Neurol Scand Suppl* 1995;161:11-22.

Poser S, Kurtzke JF: Epidemiology of MS. *Neurology* 1991;41:157-158.

Rosati G: The prevalence of multiple sclerosis in the world: an update. *Neurol Sci* 2001;22:117-139.

Stein EC, Schiffer RB, Hall WJ, et al: Multiple sclerosis and the workplace: report of an industry-based cluster. *Neurology* 1987;37:1672-1677.

Wingerchuk DM, Weinshenker BG: Multiple sclerosis: epidemiology, genetics, classification, natural history, and clinical outcome measures. *Neuroimaging Clin N Am* 2000;10:611-624.

Chapter 2

Clinical Features and Disease Course

The clinical course of multiple sclerosis (MS) is divided into categories according to neurologic symptoms as they develop over time. The commonly accepted disease classification for MS was developed by consensus among MS experts (Table 2-1).

Most patients evolve through stages, beginning with a clinically isolated syndrome (CIS), moving into relapsing-remitting MS (RRMS), and then evolving to a pattern called secondary progressive MS. This process is depicted in Figure 2-1.

Clinically Isolated Syndrome

This term refers to the initial clinical presentation of MS. Most commonly, patients presenting with MS have optic neuritis, transverse myelitis, a brainstem or cerebellar syndrome, or (less commonly), a hemispheric syndrome (eg, hemiparesis). The onset symptoms evolve over the course of a few days to a week, stabilize, and then improve over the course of weeks to a few months. As seen in Figure 2-1, the most common age at presentation is in the early 30s.

Relapsing-Remitting Multiple Sclerosis

Patients are given a definite diagnosis of RRMS when they have experienced a relapse following recovery from a CIS. Repeated relapses followed by remission is the most common clinical pattern of MS in patients under 40 years of age. Figure 2-1 shows the recurrent focal neurologic symptoms and signs occurring over 20-year period. Symp-

Table 2-1: Multiple Sclerosis Clinical Categories

Disease Category	Explanation
Clinically isolated syndromes (CIS)	The first episode of inflammatory demyelination. Patients are at high risk of developing RRMS if they have multiple brain lesions on the MRI scan
Relapsing-remitting (RRMS)	Episodes of acute worsening with recovery and a stable course between relapses
Secondary progressive MS (SPMS)	Gradual neurologic deterioration with or without superimposed acute relapses in a patient who previously had RRMS
Primary progressive MS (PPMS)*	Gradual, nearly continuous neurologic deterioration from onset of symptoms

*A less common pattern is progressive-relapsing MS (PRMS), defined as gradual neurologic deterioration from onset but with subsequent superimposed relapses.

toms range in severity and result from involvement of any part of the brain, spinal cord, or optic nerves, resulting in marked clinical heterogeneity. Common relapse symptoms include blurred vision, paresthesias or sensory loss, weakness, ataxia, diplopia, and vertigo. These symptoms and their associated signs evolve over 24 to 72 hours, stabilize for a few days, and then improve spontaneously during a period of 4 to 8 weeks. As indicated in Figure 2-1,

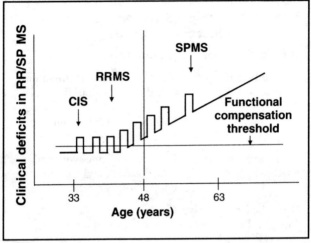

Figure 2-1: Clinical course of relapsing multiple sclerosis.

symptoms and signs commonly remit fully, but as the disease duration lengthens, incomplete recovery is more the rule. This can leave the patient with increasing neurologic deficits. Old symptoms may recur, with or without new ones, and with time it becomes difficult to determine whether the symptom flare represents a new relapse or a worsening of existing disease.

Secondary Progressive Multiple Sclerosis

Many patients with an initial RRMS course progress into a clinical pattern of progressive neurologic disability. This situation affects at least 50% of patients, and some studies suggest a much higher rate given a long enough follow-up interval. Most commonly, this pattern emerges 15 to 20 years after the initial symptoms of MS, usually between ages 45 and 55 years. A patient with secondary progressive MS (SPMS) may still experience relapses but does not stabilize between them. Rather, the predominant clinical pattern is one of continued clinical worsening. As

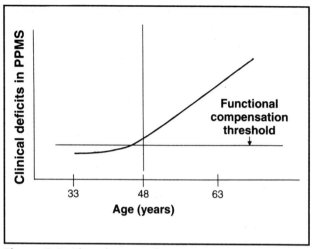

Figure 2-2: Clinical course of primary progressive MS.

time passes, relapses become less discrete, and the pattern becomes one of continued worsening without relapses. It is difficult to precisely date the time of conversion to SPMS; dating is usually fixed in retrospect. Once a patient progresses to the SPMS pattern, continued deterioration is the rule. The pathogenic mechanisms underlying conversion from RRMS to SPMS are poorly understood, but a likely possibility is the accumulation of irreversible axonal injury.

Primary Progressive Multiple Sclerosis

In approximately 15% of patients, the disease is characterized by steady worsening from the onset of symptoms (Figure 2-2). These patients tend to be older than 40 years of age at presentation, and have difficulty precisely dating the onset of symptoms. Commonly, these patients present with progressive gait disorder; leg clumsiness and spasticity are usually present. Less commonly, patients with primary progressive MS (PPMS) come to the clinician's attention because of progressive cerebellar, visual, or cognitive deficits.

Patients with PPMS have less tissue inflammation on histopathologic assessment and less cerebrospinal fluid (CSF) inflammation compared with RRMS or SPMS patients. This fact raises the question of the relationship between PPMS and other forms of MS. Ultimately, making the biologic distinction between SPMS and PPMS will require etiologic and genetic understanding of the disease.

Progressive-Relapsing Multiple Sclerosis

According to the current classification, progressive-relapsing MS (PRMS) is the term used for the patient with progressive disease from symptom onset who subsequently experiences one or more relapses. This is probably another form of SPMS without clinically apparent relapses in the early stages of disease.

Uncommon Clinical Patterns of Multiple Sclerosis

Acute Progressive Multiple Sclerosis (Marburg's Disease)

The patient with no history of MS who develops acute or subacute progressive neurologic deterioration leading to severe disability within days to months may have Marburg's disease. The patient may deteriorate steadily to a quadriplegic obtunded state with death because of intercurrent infection, aspiration, or respiratory failure. Postmortem studies have documented inflammation in the optic nerves, optic chiasma, cerebral hemispheres, and spinal cord.

Neuromyelitis Optica (Devic's Disease)

Neuromyelitis optica is a clinical syndrome consisting of optic neuritis and transverse myelitis, occurring either simultaneously or separated by only a brief interval in a person without prior evidence of MS. Postmortem studies suggest pathologic differences from typical MS. Recent immunologic studies suggest the presence of pathogenic auto-antibodies that bind to antigens in the spinal cord. Similar antibodies were not observed in patients with typical MS.

Table 2-2: Common Presenting Symptoms of Multiple Sclerosis

Symptom	Percentage*
Visual loss	49%
Weakness	43%
Paresthesias	41%
Incoordination	23%
Genitourinary/bowel	10%
Cerebral	4%

*Total adds up to more than 100 because some patients had multiple symptoms in this series. Poser et al, *J Neurol Sci* 1979;40:159-168.

Signs and Symptoms of Multiple Sclerosis

Multiple sclerosis usually presents with neurologic symptoms and signs referable to the optic nerve, pyramidal tract, posterior column, cerebellum, or brain stem. Patients in the older age group more commonly present with slowly progressive myelopathy, usually manifest as a walking problem. Spastic paraparesis, gait instability, and bladder impairment usually exist. In a large group of MS patients studied at the University of Western Ontario in the 1970s, approximately 30% presented with visual symptoms, 30% with sensory symptoms, 20% with gait or balance disturbance, and the remaining 20% with less common presentations (Table 2-2). Symptoms and signs that emerge as the disease proceeds are listed in Table 2-3. In general, as the disease progresses, new symptoms and signs appear, old symptoms and signs recur, and residual symptoms or impairments increase.

Table 2-3: Common Symptoms and Signs in Multiple Sclerosis Patients

Symptoms	Signs	Comment
Visual blurring, central visual loss, eye pain	Diminished acuity, central scotoma, deafferented pupil	Syndrome of optic neuritis, usually seen early in the disease
Diplopia, oscillopsia	Internuclear ophthalmoplegia, more rarely other oculomotor weakness, ocular dysmetria, or flutter	May be associated with nausea, vertigo, or other brain stem signs
Loss of dexterity, weakness, tightness, pain	Upper motor neuron signs affecting legs early in disease, arms later	Develops in most MS patients over time
Shaking, imbalance	Intention tremor, dysmetria, dysarthria, trunk or head titubation	Occurs in about 30% of patients; may be predominant manifestation in certain patients
Paresthesias, loss of sensation	Decreased vibration and position sense in legs more than arms; decreased fine sensation in hands	Sensory symptoms often painful and distressing

Symptoms	Signs	Comment
Inability to concentrate or learn; distractibility	Diminished concentration, processing speed, or verbal learning	May be subtle or inapparent clinically, but may have severe impact on patient and family; dementia in <10% of patients
Emotional lability or pathologic laughing and weeping	Episodic crying or laughing	Distressing to patient; may not be related to the patient's underlying mood
Depression		Commonly unrecognized or underestimated
Fatigue		Disabling in many MS patients; does not correlate with severity of motor signs
Pain		Very common, many causes
Urinary urgency, hesitancy, incontinence	Requires urodynamic testing to characterize	May be complicated by intercurrent urinary tract infection

Visual Disturbances

Visual disturbances, resulting from inflammation in the optic nerves, are among the most common symptoms of MS. Approximately 80% of patients experience visual disturbances at some time during the disease course. Visual disturbances can be in the form of optic neuritis, abnormal eye movements, double or blurred vision, or color distortion.

Optic Neuritis

Optic neuritis is the most common presenting symptom of MS. Acute optic neuritis manifests as monocular loss of central vision with eye pain. Vision loss occurs during a few hours to days, and ranges from mild to severe. Some patients notice loss of color perception. Pain commonly precedes or accompanies vision loss, and is worse with eye movement. Some patients report generalized headaches with vision loss. Optic neuritis usually begins in one eye; it is bilateral in less than 10% of cases. On examination, central vision loss can be demonstrated with bedside testing. The patient will report that parts of the examiner's face are blurred or missing. Patients with unilateral optic neuritis respond to a direct light stimulus with pupil dilation, but the affected pupil constricts on illumination of the unaffected eye. This is termed an 'afferent pupillary defect,' or Marcus Gunn pupil. Involvement of the optic nerve behind the eye is the rule, and fundoscopic examination is normal in that situation. When the optic nerve head is affected, the optic disc is congested and swollen, resembling papilledema. This is termed 'papillitis.' Less commonly, usually in older patients, optic nerve involvement manifests as slowly progressive, asymmetric, painless vision loss.

Abnormal Eye Movements

These movements occur frequently in MS and relate to lesions in the central oculomotor, vestibular, or cerebellar pathways. The most common abnormality is impaired smooth pursuit movements, or impaired saccadic movement. Pathologic lateral gaze nystagmus is also common, as is internuclear ophthalmoplegia (INO). The hallmark of an INO is impaired adduction on the side of the brain stem lesion, with lateral gaze nystagmus in the abducting eye; the paretic eye adducts normally with accommodation. Ocular dysmetria, flutter, or conjugate gaze paralysis are less common. Patients are unaware of saccadic movement, the most common oculomotor abnormality. Saccadic movement is nonspecific, however, and may be caused by many diseases, by sedative or antiepileptic drugs, or by normal aging or sleep deprivation. Ocular dysmetria or flutter is usually associated with cerebellar disease.

Spastic Weakness

The upper motor neuron syndrome is the most common motor abnormality in MS. It consists of impaired motor control, spasticity, weakness, exaggerated tendon stretch reflexes, and extensor plantar responses. Weakness affects the legs earlier than the arms in the course of disease. Paraparesis is common, spastic hemiparesis or monoparesis less common. In younger patients, an acute relapse causes the subacute onset of spastic weakness that improves during weeks to months. In older patients, slowly progressive, asymmetric paraparesis is the rule. Early on, the patient reports difficulty with motor endurance and problems with stressed gait maneuvers such as running, jumping, or walking on uneven surfaces. Over time, the problem progresses to frank functional impairment. Later in the disease, arm weakness ensues, often years after legs have become severely weakened. Initially, patients report asymmetric loss of hand dexterity and stiffness; weakness ensues later on. Leg weakness predominantly affects hip flexors, hamstrings, and ankle dorsiflexors; arm weakness most commonly affects hand intrinsic muscles, finger and wrist extensors, triceps, and deltoids. In earlier stages of the disease, weakness is evident only in the hip flexors and hand intrinsic muscles.

Some degree of spastic hypertonia usually accompanies the weakness. Symptoms include stiffness, spasms, and pain. Involuntary triple flexion or extension may occur spontaneously or may be precipitated by attempts at voluntary movement, changes in position, or cutaneous or painful stimuli. Brief, painful spasms may occur and range from infrequent to nearly continuous. Nocturnal spasms may interfere with sleep. Additionally, patients report ankle or leg clonus in the form of leg shaking or tremor. It is not uncommon to observe severe leg spasticity without significant motor weakness.

Cerebellar Signs

Axial instability ranges from slight imbalance evident when tandem walk is tested to total inability to sit unsupported. Intention tremor, dysmetria, and dysrhythmia occur in variable combination, most commonly affecting arms. Legs are less commonly affected. Intention tremor is worse with sustained posture, such as extended arms. Intention tremor is usually bilateral but asymmetric. If it was gradual in onset, the patient may be unaware it exists. Severe limb ataxia results in marked disability or even total dependence for activities of daily living. Head or trunk titubation or scanning dysarthria are occasional problems. They are usually combined with a generalized cerebellar syndrome.

Sensory Symptoms

Paresthesias affecting the extremities are common as initial symptoms and almost universal in established MS. Patients report 'pins and needles' sensations, sensory loss, or numbness. Paresthesias are commonly painful or irritating, and are described as burning, prickling, or crawling. Sensory symptoms can reflect the organization of central nervous system sensory pathways, eg, they can involve an entire limb, both extremities on one side, or both legs ascending to a spinal level. It is also common for patients to describe patches of numbness, or 'pins and needles,' in multiple areas that defy anatomic explanation.

Sensory symptoms are accompanied by loss of fine discriminating sensation. For example, two-point discrimination or graphesthesia may be diminished over affected fingertips. Posterior column signs, particularly affecting the legs, are also common and occur regularly in patients even without sensory symptoms. Loss of vibratory sensation is more severe than proprioceptive loss, although the reverse can occur. Loss of pain sensation is less common, but is observed after transverse myelitis or in the late stages of MS. Lhermitte's sign, which is a shooting electric sensation precipitated by neck flexion, may also occur. Tingling, electrical-shock-like sensation with neck flexion travels into the arms or back. Lhermitte's sign indicates cervical spinal cord disease; while common in MS with cervical cord involvement, it is not specific for MS.

Cognitive and Memory Impairment

Cognitive and memory impairment occur frequently in MS patients. Population surveys have shown that about 50% of MS patients exhibit significant impairment relative to age- and gender-matched healthy controls.

Areas of most common impairment include speed of information processing, sustained attention and concentration, and verbal learning. There is relatively little problem with language, abstract reasoning, visual spacial function, or insight. In many cases, problems are subtle and not disabling, but they may have functional consequences at work or at home, and patients, family members, and physicians frequently fail to recognize the underlying problem. Severe, dementing illness can occur with relatively little motor impairment, but this is rare. A correlation between the severity of cognitive impairment and the severity of brain disease measured by magnetic resonance imaging (MRI) has been reported. Cognitive impairment correlates poorly with the degree of motor impairment, but is undoubtedly a significant cause of disability and family distress.

Emotional Lability

Pathologic laughing and weeping occur in more than 10% of MS patients, and range from a barely noticeable tendency to giggle or tear easily through a distressing, less-common syndrome of powerful, paroxysmal emotional outbursts. Laughing or weeping may be precipitated by seemingly innocuous stimuli. The patient's emotional expression is not accompanied by a similar internal feeling. For example, patients will laugh when they do not feel happy, or cry when they do not feel sad. When asked, patients will report the discrepancy between their emotional expression and internal feelings. They may be perplexed and embarrassed by this. Pathologic laughing and weeping is categorized as a disconnection syndrome, in which descending pathways to the brain stem are disconnected, leading to the release of emotional display. It is commonly seen in the context of pseudobulbar palsy with dysarthria and dysphagia, indicating bilateral corticobulbar and corticospinal disease. The actual neural pathways involved are not known, but it is important to recognize this syndrome because the impact on the patient and family may be severe. Pathologic laughter may mask an underlying depression, which itself may be partly a reaction to the emotional incontinence.

Depression

Depression is common in MS patients, exceeding the frequency in comparative groups with other severe neurologic disease such as temporal lobe epilepsy or amyotrophic lateral sclerosis. The mechanisms of depression in MS are not completely understood, but the uncertainties related to future disease state and progression, plus loss of a sense of control over one's health, are undoubtedly factors. Suicide is a risk in some patients, so the assessing physician must consider it. Depression may be recurrent, or it may be part of a bipolar illness.

Fatigue

Fatigue may be the most common complaint of MS patients. MS fatigue is multifactorial. Undoubtedly, it may be caused by the disease itself. The presence of disabling fatigue out of proportion to physical impairments, depression, or sleep disturbance suggests this. MS fatigue usually comes on in the afternoon. It is worse with strenuous activity, or with exposure to heat. The clinician must differentiate it from normal fatigue that occurs only after extraordinary effort and from the fatigue experienced as part of depression.

Two specific syndromes are seen. Nerve fiber fatigue causes neurologic symptoms with repetitive use of the pathway. For example, vision may fail in bright light or with continuous reading, or ambulation may fail with distance walk. Short rest periods restore function in this situation. A more generalized fatigue is thought to be primarily related to MS but occurs via mechanisms that are not understood. It can take the form of overwhelming, often disabling lassitude.

Pain

In Clifford and Trotter's series of 317 MS patients, 28.8% complained of significant pain. The most common type of pain is low back, hip, or leg pain. Muscle and joint strain related to weakness or spasticity underlies much of this problem. Nerve root compression caused by intervertebral disc bulge or rupture occurs. Some patients report paroxysmal, painful paresthesias. These symptoms are described as shooting, burning, or tingling pain. Typical trigeminal neuralgia, or atypical facial pain, is caused by disease in the pontine tegmentum. Facial pain is bilateral in many cases.

Bladder Dysfunction

Bladder disturbance is the first manifestation in only a small minority of MS patients, but later in the disease it occurs in at least two thirds. Patients most commonly report urgency, frequency, and urge incontinence, but hesitancy and a sense of incomplete emptying are also common. Bladder dysfunction is important because of its severe, negative impact on the quality of life. Effective symptomatic treatments are available.

Bladder dysfunction can be divided into two categories: spastic and flaccid. Patients with flaccid bladder may fail to empty urine adequately, leading to high urinary residual volumes, and at times to frank urinary retention. Associated symptoms include urinary hesitancy, postvoid fullness or dribbling, or frank inability to initiate urination despite a feeling of fullness. Urinary retention may arise from detrusor atony, external sphincter spasm, or outlet obstruction from some other cause, such as prostatic hypertrophy. Alternatively, patients with spastic bladder may fail to properly store urine, reporting symptoms such as urgency, urge incontinence, dysuria, frequency, and nocturia. Failure to store urine may be due to detrusor hyperactivity, spontaneous detrusor spasms, or a low-capacity bladder. The correlation between bladder symptoms and the underlying pathophysiology is weak. At a minimum, the clinician must determine postvoid residual urine volume to determine if there is complete emptying. Urologic evaluation with urodynamic testing may be necessary. A major complication of bladder dysfunction is recurrent urinary tract infection. This is an indication for urologic assessment and therapy designed to eliminate infection.

Bowel Symptoms

Constipation is common and can become a major problem. Impaired postprandial colonic motor activity has been reported in MS patients with severe constipation. This problem is similar to findings in patients with thoracic spinal cord injury and probably represents autonomic dysfunction. Drugs with anticholinergic effects, such as antidepressants, or drugs for spastic bladder, may worsen constipation due to MS. Sacral sensory loss, anal sphincter atony, or fecal incontinence may also be distressing problems in patients with lumbosacral cord involvement.

Autonomic Nervous System Dysfunction

Clinicians see dependent vascular congestion or color change in the feet with moderate frequency. Vascular instability is probably due to autonomic hyperreflexia from central autonomic pathway involvement. It appears to be analogous to the increase in tendon reflexes seen in the upper motor neuron syndrome. This problem is most common in patients with moderate-to-severe paraparesis, but it may be seen in patients with relatively little motor impairment. Patients report a 'hot and cold foot syndrome' in which their feet are either pale and cold or hot and flushed, but are rarely comfortable. This symptom is most bothersome at night.

Autonomic dysfunction may also contribute to the dependent edema that frequently accompanies paraparesis and paraplegia, although the loss of normal motor activity is probably the major factor in this problem. Postural hypotension is rarely a problem in MS, and symptomatic cardiac dysfunction due to altered sympathetic or parasympathetic activity is rare. Abnormal sweating occasionally occurs but is rarely symptomatic. In rare instances, sweating abnormalities may interfere with the regulation of body temperature, particularly in advanced cases.

Sexual Dysfunction

Sexual dysfunction is common. In a population survey, 56% of women and 75% of men reported sexual problems, including fatigue, decreased sensation, decreased libido, erectile dysfunction, and a myriad of other symptoms. The sexual problems do not appear to be closely associated with the extent of motor system impairment. The natural history, frequency, etiology, and treatment for most of these disorders have not been established.

Paroxysmal Syndromes

Paroxysmal disorders include dystonic spasms, trigeminal neuralgia, paresthesias, and seizures. Dystonic spasms, or 'tonic seizures,' occur in a small proportion of patients. They consist of brief, recurrent, painful posturing in one or more limbs. The arm is most commonly involved, but tonic spasms can involve one entire side of the body. Tonic spasms are not associated with altered consciousness or with involuntary micturition, but may be associated with relatively inconspicuous distal clonic movements or writhing movements. Dystonic spasms are mostly spontaneous. Movement and cutaneous or painful stimuli may also precipitate them. Seizures occur in approximately 5% of MS patients at some point in their illness, usually taking the form of secondary, generalized tonic-clonic seizures, beginning focally. Patients with cortical and subcortical lesions on cranial MRI are more likely to have seizures. MS presents as a seizure disorder only rarely. Focal seizures are rare. Most patients with seizures are controlled with anticonvulsants.

Other Manifestations

Other disease manifestations are rare. They include aphasia, homonymous hemianopsia, gait apraxia, or involuntary movements. Nonfluent aphasia due to MS has been reported. Comprehension is spared, and the language problem tends to improve. Homonymous field cuts are uncommon but have been reported. Movement disorders in MS include dystonia, facial myokymia, myoclonus of various types, and choreoathetosis. Patients may develop gait apraxia that resembles the gait disturbance seen in normal pressure hydrocephalus.

Disease Severity and Prognostic Factors

As with other chronic diseases, severity varies among MS patients. There is debate about how often MS takes a truly benign form, and no consensus exists on how to define benign MS. A commonly cited figure is 20%: a common definition is the absence of vocational, social, or physical limitations 10 years after the first symptom. Patients with benign MS may have occasional episodes and periodic symptoms but do not follow a course of increasing impairment. Cases of optic neuritis or transverse myelitis without recurrence probably fall into this category. At the other end of the spectrum, a small minority of patients follow a malignant course with disease onset progressing to severe physical disability within a few years.

Table 2-4: Effects of Baseline MRI Scan on Prognosis in Patients With Clinically Isolated Syndrome

Outcome After 5 years	Brain Lesions by MRI	Normal Brain MRI Scan
RRMS	90%	0%
Measurable disability	52%	6%

In most patients, the disease severity is intermediate, and the illness is characterized by fluctuating and varied symptoms, a wide range of disabilities, and a course spanning decades.

Prognosis at the Time of Clinically Isolated Syndrome

The clinical features are not helpful in predicting future disease course in patients with a CIS. Disease severity measured by MRI at this stage does help, however. Fillipi et al found that patients with CIS and multiple brain lesions on cranial MRI scan at the time of presentation were more likely to develop MS and significant disability than patients who appeared clinically similar but had normal brain MRI scans (Table 2-4). Such patients have been followed for nearly 15 years, and the data indicate that those with CIS and a normal MRI scan have a relatively favorable prognosis.

On the other hand, it is highly likely that a patient presenting with a CIS and brain lesions will have another clinical relapse and will convert to definite RRMS. These patients find it useful to have some idea of how severe the disease is likely to be. Physicians find similar information useful for making therapeutic decisions. Table 2-5 lists favorable and unfavorable prognostic markers in patients with definite MS.

Table 2-5: Clinical Markers of Prognosis in Patients With Established Multiple Sclerosis*

Relatively Favorable	Relatively Unfavorable
Female	Male
Onset as relapsing-remitting MS	Onset as progressive MS
Predominant sensory symptoms or optic neuritis	Predominant motor or cerebellar signs
Complete recovery from relapse	Poor recovery from relapse
Long interval between relapses	Short interval between relapses
Long time to impaired ambulation	Short time to impaired ambulation

*With the exception of progressive MS from onset, these clinical and demographic markers are only weak predictors of future disease severity.

In one study, 71 patients with isolated syndromes were re-evaluated after an average of 14 years. Clinically definite MS had developed in 88% of those who presented with brain lesions and in 19% of those who had an initially normal brain MRI scan. The accumulation of T_2 brain lesions during the initial 5 years correlated significantly with disability at the 14-year follow-up. In another study, 163 patients with established RRMS, mean disease duration 6 years, were evaluated during a 2-year observation period and then re-evaluated 8 years later. In these patients, the amount of brain atrophy at 6 years' disease duration and the amount of brain atrophy progression between 6 and 8 years' disease duration, correlated with the degree of physical disability 8 years later. These studies indicate that MRI lesions and brain atrophy in the early stage of MS correlate with neurologic disability later on. However, the correlations are still modest, so prognosis cannot be predicted with confidence in individual patients.

Precipitating Factors
Viral Infection

Viral infection is often mentioned as a possible preceding event. However, the low incidence of the disease and the delay in diagnosis make prospective studies difficult. In prospective studies, Sibley et al found that viral infections may precipitate relapses in patients with established MS. One hundred seventy MS patients were studied longitudinally. The 'at risk' period was defined as the period from 2 weeks before to 5 weeks after clinical viral infections. The risk of a clinical MS relapse was threefold higher during 'at risk' periods compared with periods more distant from viral infections. Twenty-seven percent of relapses in Sibley's study were correlated with viral infections.

Anderson followed 60 MS patients with similar methodology. During 4-week 'at risk' periods, there was a significant excess of MS relapses, with a relative risk of 1.3. The Anderson study suggested that adenovirus infection was associated with severe MS relapses.

Vaccination

Vaccination has been suggested as a possible precipitating event for MS, but so far prospective studies have failed to establish a relationship between vaccination and relapses. A recent study failed to demonstrate a relationship between influenza vaccination and acute relapses.

Traumatic Injury

Traumatic injury has been suggested as a possible precipitating event. Most neurologists have seen cases in which the first attack of MS followed significant brain or spinal cord injury, or where established MS worsened after traumatic injury. Epidemiologic studies have failed to demonstrate any association between onset of MS and head injury or spinal disk surgery, or any evidence that traumatic injury accelerated disease progression in patients with established MS. It remains possible that traumatic injury can precipitate disease onset or worsen MS in susceptible individuals, but this is entirely conjectural.

Pregnancy

The relationship of pregnancy to acute attacks of MS has been reviewed. Fertility does not appear to be significantly affected by MS and the disease itself has little effect on the course of pregnancy or labor. Pregnancy is associated with a decreased risk of acute attacks, but the postpartum period is associated with a high risk for relapse. The risk of an acute attack in the first 3 months postpartum has been estimated to be between 20% and 40%. The decreased relapse rate during pregnancy is probably related to a family of immunosuppressive hormones of fetal, placental, or maternal origin. Overall, pregnancy probably has little effect on the course of the disease.

Common Patterns of Disease

Clinical manifestations in patients with well-established MS are an admixture of optic nerve, oculomotor, pyramidal, cerebellar, and posterior column involvement. The specific manifestations usually include vision loss, diplopia, oscillopsia, gait disturbance, spastic weakness, ataxia, and sensory symptoms. A sizable minority of patients can be categorized into common clinical patterns.

Myelopathy

Patients with myelopathy usually have onset after 35 years of age, commonly in the fourth or fifth decade of life. They present with an insidiously progressive gait disorder or with a monoparesis first involving one leg and then spreading to involve both. Bladder disturbance and sensory involvement commonly accompany the other features. The diagnosis can be difficult or even impossible, particularly when patients have no evidence of disseminated disease. Evoked potential testing and/or brain imaging will often (but by no means always) provide evidence for a separate lesion. CSF testing gives abnormal results in only 50% of these patients. The clinician must be vigilant in ruling out the presence of structural disease of the spinal cord.

Cerebellar Syndrome

Patients with cerebellar syndrome frequently have prominent axial, appendicular, and oculomotor cerebellar signs. Other neurologic signs may be relatively subtle, so that the illness may closely mimic heredofamilial cerebellar degeneration. Clinicians must be certain to rule out structural disease in the posterior fossa, however. Most patients with this form of disease also have typical CSF abnormalities.

Optic Neuropathy

Progressive vision loss without other manifestations has been described in MS. Of principal concern are compressive lesions at the base of the brain.

Cognitive Impairment

In some patients, progressive cognitive impairment appears to be an early and predominant manifestation. Again, caution must be exercised in ruling out alternative diagnoses.

Suggested Readings

Amato MP, Ponziani G: A prospective study on the prognosis of multiple sclerosis. *J Neurol Sci* 2000;21:S831-S838.

Brex PA, Ciccarelli O, O'Riordan JI, et al: A longitudinal study of abnormalities on MRI and disability from multiple sclerosis. *N Engl J Med* 2002;346:158-164.

Clifford DB, Trotter JL: Pain in multiple sclerosis. *Arch Neurol* 1984;41:1270-1272.

Confavreux C, Vukusic S, Moreau T, et al: Relapses and progression of disability in multiple sclerosis. *N Engl J Med* 2000;343:1430-1438.

Cook SD: Trauma does not precipitate multiple sclerosis. *Arch Neurol* 2000;57:1077-1078.

Currie R: Spasticity: a common symptom of multiple sclerosis. *Nurs Stand* 2001;15:47-52.

Lublin FD, Reingold SC: Defining the clinical course of multiple sclerosis: results of an international survey. National Multiple Sclerosis Society (USA) Advisory Committee on Clinical Trials of New Agents in Multiple Sclerosis. *Neurology* 1996;46:907-911.

Holland N: Primary care management of multiple sclerosis. *Adv Nurse Pract* 1999;7:26-32.

McDonald WI: Relapse, remission, and progression in multiple sclerosis. *N Engl J Med* 2000;343:1486-1487.

Poser S, Wikstrom J, Bauer HJ: Clinical data and the identification of special forms of multiple sclerosis in 1,271 cases studied with a standardized documentation system. *J Neurol Sci* 1979;40:159-168.

Rao SM: Neuropsychology of multiple sclerosis: a critical review. *J Clin Exp Neuropsychol* 1986;8:503-542.

Schiffer RB, Caine ED, Bamford KA, et al: Depressive episodes in patients with multiple sclerosis. *Am J Psychiatry* 1983;140:1498-1500.

Weinshenker BG, Ebers GC: The natural history of multiple sclerosis. *Can J Neurol Sci* 1987;14:255-261.

Weinshenker BG: Neuromyelitis optica: what it is and what it might be. *Lancet* 2003;361;889-890.

Chapter 3

Diagnosis and Differential Diagnosis

Accurate diagnosis of multiple sclerosis (MS) is critically important because effective disease-modifying therapy is available (see Chapter 8). In the relapsing stage of MS, disease-modifying therapy reduces the frequency and severity of relapses, delays disability progression, and significantly reduces new magnetic resonance imaging (MRI) lesions. A strong feeling exists among MS experts that early diagnosis is important so that disease-modifying drug therapy can be initiated early, when it appears to be more effective. Accurate diagnosis also removes uncertainty, allows informed planning, and contributes to an improved sense of well being for the patient. This chapter reviews diagnostic criteria and tests for MS, examines the differential diagnosis, and lists clues to an incorrect diagnosis that should prompt targeted diagnostic testing.

The diagnosis is strongly suggested in an otherwise healthy 33-year-old woman who has experienced two or more acute episodes of central nervous system (CNS) dysfunction (eg, optic neuritis that resolved, followed later by an episode of gait ataxia, and later by an episode of transient leg weakness). The diagnosis in this case is confirmed by clinical deficits related to CNS disease, typical MRI lesions, and cerebrospinal fluid (CSF) changes suggesting MS.

The diagnosis is often not so straightforward, however, and the rate of inaccurate diagnosis ranges from 5% to

10%. Inaccurate diagnoses fall into two categories. Patients with a different neurologic disease may be labeled as having MS. Tumors and other mass lesions are suspected when clinical features could be caused by a single-site lesion in the CNS. Mass lesions should be ruled out with MRI. Degenerative, infectious, or neoplastic diseases can masquerade as MS. They should be considered in patients with steadily progressive deterioration from disease onset. Spinocerebellar degeneration, B_{12} deficiency, human T-cell lymphotrophic virus type 1 (HTLV-1) myelopathy, and multicentric brain lymphoma are the most common conditions incorrectly diagnosed as MS in this group. CNS lupus and small vessel cerebrovascular disease may be clinically similar to relapsing MS. Normal CSF, atypical cranial MRI findings, and clinical features associated with the underlying disease are clues. Secondly, patients with nonspecific neurologic symptoms such as fatigue, tingling, or dizziness may be incorrectly diagnosed with MS. Normal imaging and CSF tests and disability out of proportion to objective findings raise doubts about the diagnosis of MS.

Diagnostic Criteria

Even though highly characteristic MRI findings come close to being diagnostic (see Chapter 4), there is no accepted definitive diagnostic test for MS. Consequently, diagnostic criteria are used to minimize the likelihood of misdiagnosis. The first widely applied diagnostic criteria—Schumacher criteria (Table 3-1)—laid out critical clinical principles that persist now. Schumacher criteria recognized that MS was a chronic, active disease process involving white matter and affecting young people. Objective neurologic deficits were required to document lesion dissemination over time and in location within the CNS. The criteria also recognized two subtypes of disease, relapsing and progressive. Schumacher criteria used only clinical data, however, and were formulated in an

Table 3-1: Schumacher Criteria for Definite Multiple Sclerosis

- 10 to 50 years of age
- Central nervous system white matter disease
- Lesions disseminated in time and space
- Objective abnormalities on examination
- Time course: attacks lasting more than 24 hours, spaced 1 month apart; or slow or stepwise progression for 6 months
- No better explanation
- Diagnosis made by a competent neurologist

era without sensitive imaging procedures. Schumacher criteria are useful but it is often not possible to diagnose MS in the early stages using these clinical guidelines.

The Poser criteria were proposed in 1983 to incorporate laboratory testing in MS diagnosis. MRI was rapidly becoming an important aspect of diagnostic testing in suspected MS. The Poser criteria maintained the general concepts from Schumacher, but allowed second lesions to be documented by MRI scan or evoked potential testing. The Poser criteria also referred to CSF testing for oligoclonal bands (OCBs), elevated immunoglobulin G (IgG) index, or increased CNS IgG synthesis. This provides laboratory support for the diagnosis.

The Poser criteria were developed for research studies, and clinicians found them too cumbersome and complex for routine clinical practice. Recently, an international task force published the current criteria in 2001 (Tables 3-2 and 3-3). These criteria place less emphasis on sensory evoked potentials or CSF analysis, and relatively more emphasis on MRI changes.

Table 3-2: International Diagnostic Criteria

Clinical Presentation	Additional Data Needed for MS Diagnosis
Two or more relapses; objective clinical evidence of 2 or more lesions	None
Two or more relapses; objective clinical evidence of 1 lesion	Dissemination in space by MRI* or 2 or more MRI-detected lesions consistent with MS plus positive CSF, or await further clinical attack implicating a different site
One relapse; objective clinical evidence of 2 or more lesions	Dissemination in time by MRI** or second clinical relapse
One relapse; objective clinical evidence of 1 lesion (monosymptomatic presentation; clinically isolated syndrome)	Dissemination in space by MRI* or 2 or more MRI-detected lesions consistent with MS plus positive CSF and dissemination in time by MRI** or second clinical relapse
Insidious neurologic progression suggestive of MS	Positive CSF and dissemination in space by MRI* and dissemination in time by MRI** or clinical progression for at least 1 year

Adapted from McDonald WI et al, *Ann Neurol* 2001; 50:121-127.
*Table 3-3
**Table 3-4

> **Table 3-3: International Panel Criteria for Abnormal Magnetic Resonance Imaging Scan (3 of the Following)**
>
> - One gadolinium-enhancing lesion, or 9 T_2-hyperintense lesions if there is no gadolinium-enhancing lesion
> - At least 1 infratentorial lesion
> - At least 1 juxtacortical lesion
> - At least 3 periventricular lesions
>
> Adapted from McDonald WI et al, *Ann Neurol* 2001; 50:121-127.

The International Panel Criteria maintain the principles from the Schumacher criteria—dissemination of lesions in space and time—but allow the use of MRI scans to document this. There are two areas of controversy related to the International Panel Criteria. First, many MS experts believe it is possible to diagnose MS at the time the patient presents with a clinically isolated syndrome, provided there are multiple, appropriately placed brain lesions on the MRI scan. The International Panel Criteria do not recognize a diagnosis at the first clinical presentation, instead requiring dissemination in time by repeat MRI scans showing new lesions (Table 3-4). The second area of controversy is in the diagnosis of primary progressive MS. The International Panel Criteria require CSF findings of increased IgG or OCBs. However, in a series of more than 700 patients with primary progressive MS (PPMS) entered into a clinical trial, nearly 1 of 5 had normal CSF findings. These patients were clinically indistinguishable from the patients with OCBs, except for their MRI findings. The CSF negative patients

Table 3-4: International Panel Criteria for Dissemination of Lesions in Time

- If a first scan occurs 3 months or more after the onset of the clinical event, the presence of a gadolinium-enhancing lesion is sufficient to demonstrate dissemination in time, provided that it is not at the site implicated in the original clinical event. If there is no enhancing lesion at this time, a follow-up scan is required at least 3 months after the initial scan. A new T_2- or gadolinium-enhancing lesion at this time then fulfills the criterion for dissemination in time.

- If the first scan is performed less than 3 months after the onset of the clinical event, a second scan done 3 months or more after the clinical event showing a new gadolinium-enhancing lesion provides sufficient evidence for dissemination in time. However, if no enhancing lesion is seen at this second scan, a further scan not less than 3 months after the first scan that shows a new T_2 lesion or an enhancing lesion will suffice.

Adapted from McDonald WI et al, *Ann Neurol* 2001; 50:121-127.

had less gadolinium enhancement and lower T_2 lesion burden on cranial MRI scans, but similar amounts of brain atrophy. The need for CSF testing in a patient who otherwise appears to have PPMS remains controversial.

Laboratory Investigation

The International Panel Criteria indicate that a patient with two or more relapses, and objective clinical evidence of two or more lesions, requires no further testing. How-

Table 3-5: Laboratory Testing of Multiple Sclerosis

Magnetic Resonance Imaging Scans

- Cranial (*every case*)
  - To diagnose MS
- Spinal cord (*as appropriate*)
  - To document lesions
  - To R/O cord AVM, tumor, or disc

Blood Tests

- Screening labs (*every case*)
  - ANA, B_{12}, CBC, ESR
- Specific Dx (*as appropriate*)
  - Serology for collagen vascular disease or vasculitis
  - Serology for Lyme/syphilis, HIV, HTLV-1
  - Thyroid function testing (R/O hypothyroidism)
  - Paraneoplastic syndromes (eg, anti-Hu)
  - Sarcoidosis
  - VLCFA (adrenoleukodystrophy)

Cerebrospinal Fluid (as appropriate)

- Confirm MS Dx (OCB, increased IgG or kappa chains, mononuclear pleocytosis)
- Exclude tumor or infection

Sensory Evoked Potentials (as appropriate)

- Used to document and localize lesions in visual, auditory, or somatosensory pathways

Table 3-6: MRI Features That Strongly Suggest Multiple Sclerosis

- ≥ 4 white matter lesions (≥ 3 mm)
- 3 white matter lesions, 1 periventricular
- Lesions ≥ 6 mm diameter
- Ovoid lesions, perpendicular to ventricles
- Corpus callosum lesions
- Brain stem lesions
- Ring appearance on contrast MRI

ever, many experts believe that every MS patient should have testing to support the diagnosis and rule out alternatives. At a minimum, this involves a cranial MRI scan. In addition to diagnostic support, the cranial MRI scan provides information about disease severity and activity (Chapter 4).

The exact composition of laboratory testing and its sequence depend on clinical features. Table 3-5 provides an approach to diagnostic tests. Brain MRI is abnormal in 90% to 95% of MS patients, but the figure may be lower on initial evaluation. The features listed in Table 3-6 strongly suggest MS. In a patient with typical clinical features and the MRI features listed in Table 3-6, more extensive testing may not be necessary. Many experts would argue that such a patient does not need lumbar puncture for CSF analysis.

MRI lesions from brain vascular disease become increasingly common after 50 years of age, so the specificity of MRI scan decreases. Spinal MRI should be done when the cranial MRI is negative but suspicion of MS remains. Spinal MRI may also be helpful in an older patient with nonspecific cranial MRI abnormalities, because age-related MRI lesions do not occur in the spinal cord.

Table 3-7: CSF Features That Support a Diagnosis of Multiple Sclerosis

- Normal protein, glucose
- 5 to 20 mononuclear cells/μL (lymphocytes, monocytes)
- Intrathecal IgG synthesis
    - IgG index, IgG synthesis rate
    - Oligoclonal bands
    - Free kappa light chains

Spinal MRI shows abnormalities in more than 50% of patients with established MS.

Blood work is used for conditions that masquerade as MS, or could confound the diagnosis. A reasonable panel includes antinuclear antibody (ANA), B_{12} level, complete blood count (CBC), and erythrocyte sedimentation rate (ESR). Other tests listed in Table 3-5 should be used, depending on the clinical circumstances. A patient presenting with progressive myelopathy should be checked with human immunodeficiency virus (HIV) and HTLV-1 titers, thyroid function testing, and very long chain fatty acids. Patients presenting with a cerebellar syndrome should be screened for paraneoplastic syndromes.

Lumbar puncture for CSF testing should be done in all patients with progressive disease from onset, with atypical MRI features, or with atypical clinical features. Typical CSF findings (Table 3-7) strongly support the diagnosis of MS, but are not entirely specific. Elevated CSF protein levels are not caused by MS, so an alternative explanation is needed (eg, diabetes, hypothyroidism). Similarly, abnormal glucose levels must be explained by another disease (eg, sarcoidosis). Cell counts greater than 50 per μL, or the presence of polymorphonuclear cells require testing for alternative diagnoses (eg, tumor or infection). Testing for intrathecal IgG synthesis or OCBs requires that a matching serum sample accompany the CSF to the laboratory. OCBs and increased intrathecal synthesis of IgG are not entirely specific for MS; they have been reported in patients with infections, paraneoplastic syndromes, and intracranial tumor.

Somatosensory evoked potentials are sometimes valuable to detect silent lesions in the optic nerves, or somatosensory or auditory pathways. They are used to confirm dissemination within the CNS or to determine whether a symptom is accompanied by objective neurologic deficits when the neurologic examination is normal. Patients with otherwise typical MS do not require a battery of somatosensory evoked potential tests. This has been largely supplanted by MRI scans.

Clinically isolated syndromes that may represent the onset of MS include isolated optic neuritis, acute transverse myelopathy, and acute brain stem syndrome. In these situations, MRI and CSF findings suggesting MS place the patient at high risk for subsequent relapse and new MRI lesions. Such a patient should be treated with disease-modifying drug therapy (see Chapter 8), or observed with clinical and MRI follow-up.

Acute disseminating encephalomyelitis (ADEM) is a rare condition, often mistaken for MS. ADEM presents as multicentric CNS dysfunction accompanied by fever, meningeal signs, altered consciousness, and disseminated acute brain lesions by MRI scan. The onset is often acute, sometimes subacute. Significant recovery is common, but often there are residual deficits. It is almost always a monophasic disease.

Clues to Misdiagnosis and Differential Diagnosis

Atypical features—the so-called 'red flags'—raise concerns about the accuracy of the diagnosis (Table 3-8).

Table 3-8: Features Suggesting Misdiagnosis of Multiple Sclerosis

Red Flag	Concern
Normal examination	Is there any evidence of definable neurologic disease?
Lack of dissemination in space	Is there a mass or structural lesion?

Genetic 'red flag'
  Prominent family history
  Early age onset
	Is this a genetic disorder (eg, mitochondrial disease)?

Clues to degenerative disease
  Progressive from onset
  Normal CSF
  Normal brain MRI
  Peripheral neuropathy
  Dementia, seizures, aphasia
  Fasciculations, extrapyramidal features
  Myelopathy without bladder involvement
	Is this spinocerebellar degeneration, ALS, multiple system atrophy, or other neurodegenerative disease?

Clues to vascular disease
  Atypical MRI
  Acute onset
  Hemiparesis, homonymous field cuts
	Is this small vessel cerebrovascular disease, vasculitis, or complicated migraine?

Patients without neurologic findings, and with normal cranial MRI and CSF tests in all likelihood do not have MS, though it is common for such patients who experience nonspecific symptoms such as fatigue and paresthesias to cling to this diagnosis. A clinical picture consistent with a solitary lesion in the CNS should prompt appropriate imaging studies to rule out tumor or mass lesion. The most common scenario in this category is a middle-aged or older patient with paraparesis who is diagnosed with MS, has nonspecific cranial MRI findings, and is found to have cervical spine disease with cord compression, or a spinal cord tumor. Clues to degenerative diseases or vascular disease are listed in Table 3-8.

Suggested Readings

Gasperini C: Differential diagnosis in multiple sclerosis. *Neurol Sci* 2001;22(suppl 2):S93-S97.

McDonald WI, Compston A, Edan G, et al: Recommended diagnostic criteria for multiple sclerosis: guidelines from the International Panel on the diagnosis of multiple sclerosis. *Ann Neurol* 2001;50:121-127.

McFarland HF: The emerging role of MRI in multiple sclerosis and the new diagnostic criteria. *Mult Scler* 2002;8:71-72.

Poser CM: MRI of spinal cord in multiple sclerosis. *Lancet* 1993;341:1025.

Poser CM, Paty DW, Scheinberg L, et al: New diagnostic criteria for multiple sclerosis: guidelines for research protocols. *Ann Neurol* 1983;13:227-231.

Rudick RA, Schiffer RB, Schwetz KM, et al: Multiple sclerosis. The problem of incorrect diagnosis. *Arch Neurol* 1986;43:578-583.

Schumacher GA: Multiple sclerosis. *Arch Neurol* 1966;14:571-573.

Thompson AJ, Montalban X, Barkhof F, et al: Diagnostic criteria for primary progressive multiple sclerosis: a position paper. *Ann Neurol* 2000;47:831-835.

Trojano M, Paolicelli D: The differential diagnosis of multiple sclerosis: classification and clinical features of relapsing and progressive neurological syndromes. *Neurol Sci* 2001;22(suppl 2):S98-S102.

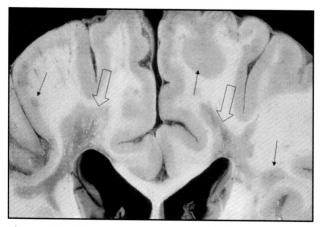

Figure 5-1: Gross appearance of the MS brain at autopsy: coronal section of a brain from an MS patient. Note the following: (1) enlarged lateral ventricles, (2) bilateral periventricular (dark brown) confluent plaques (open arrows), (3) scattered (dark brown) plaques in the hemispheric white matter bilaterally (small arrows).

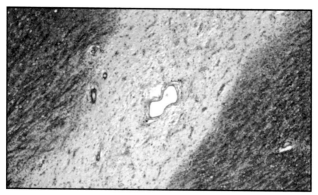

Figure 5-2: Demyelination in an MS plaque: myelin stain of an MS lesion. Blue is myelin. Note the loss of myelin, surrounding a central blood vessel, with sharply demarcated plaque borders.

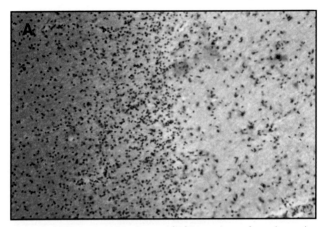

Figure 5-3: Acute MS plaque. **(A)** Note loss of myelin to the right, evident by pale staining, and intact myelin to the left, indicated by more intense staining. The intact area is separated

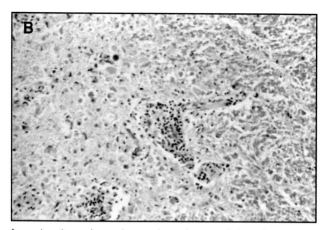

from the demyelinated zone by a hypercellular plaque margin. **(B)** Note perivascular inflammatory infiltrate, consisting of lymphocytes and monocytes, present at the plaque margin.

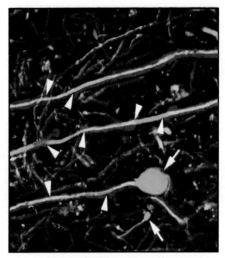

Figure 5-4: Axonal transection in acute MS lesion: confocal microscopy from an active MS lesion. Myelin is stained red, and axons are green. The figure shows demyelination affecting all three fibers in the plane of the section. In the top two axons, myelin is missing in segments (between arrow heads). The bottom fiber is transected, and the transected end is swollen (arrow).

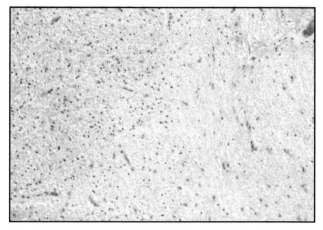

Figure 5-5: Chronic inactive plaque. Note reduced cellularity to the right. These plaques are characterized by astrocytic gliosis, lack of inflammatory infiltrate, and absence of active demyelination. They presumably represent old, 'burned out' lesions.

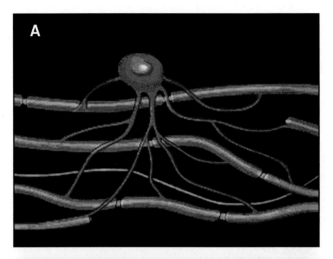

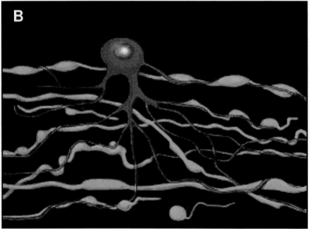

Figure 5-6: (A) An artist's rendition of a normal oligodendro-cyte myelinating CNS internodes. Myelin is shown in red, CNS axons in green. **(B)** A typical example of an oligodendrocyte observed within an MS lesion. The oligodendrocyte processes contact axons but do not lay down compact myelin. After the work by Trapp et al, *N Engl J Med*.

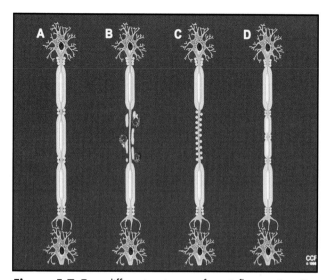

Figure 5-7: Two different outcomes from inflammation. Demyelination is shown in panel 1 and axonal transection in panel 2. At the time of inflammatory demyelination **(1B)**, axonal conduction fails because of the acute disruption of myelin and axonal function. After inflammation subsides, sodium channels redistribute along the demyelinated axon **(1C)**, and conduction is restored. Along with this process, symptoms improve and patients recover from relapse. Some degree of remyelination occurs, although the myelin internodes are short and myelin thickness is diminished **(1D)**. **(Continued on next page)**

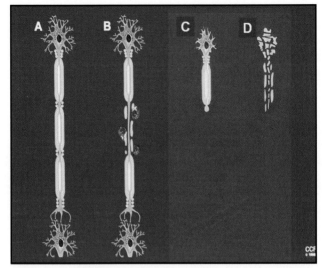

Figure 5-7 (continued): Some axons are transected at the time of inflammatory demyelination **(2C)**, leading to axonal degeneration **(2C, 2D)**. Axons affected in this way will not recover function. This process is subclinical until a critical threshold of axonal damage is exceeded. Further injury at that stage leads to progressive loss of neurologic function.

Chapter 4

Magnetic Resonance Imaging

Magnetic resonance imaging (MRI) has transformed diagnosis, management, and clinical research in multiple sclerosis (MS) in the 20 years since it was introduced to clinical medicine. Table 4-1 lists the main uses for MRI scanning—to determine diagnosis, prognosis, disease activity, and severity, and to monitor the course of the disease.

Cranial computerized tomography (CT) may reveal small lesions that are enhanced following conventional or high-volume contrast administration; hypodense, non-enhancing lesions in the periventricular white matter; or ventricular enlargement. The enhanced lesions are acute and lose their enhanced characteristics after a few weeks. Cranial CT scanning may also identify mass lesions or infarction. Cranial MRI scanning has supplanted cranial CT because the MRI scan is much more sensitive. In one comparison of CT to MRI, CT identified 19 lesions, but MRI identified 131 lesions in the same patients. At present, MRI is the imaging test of choice, and there is no reason to obtain a cranial CT scan in a patient with suspected MS.

There are three types of MS lesions, as listed in Table 4-2. One type, T_2 lesions, appears as areas of high signal in the cerebral white matter on T_2-weighted images (Figure 4-1). These T_2 lesions are typically seen within the body of the corpus callosum, extending from it like fingers reaching into the adjacent cerebral white matter.

Table 4-1: Use of Magnetic Resonance Imaging in Multiple Sclerosis

*Diagnosis**

Complements clinical assessment by providing evidence for characteristic MRI lesions and change over time

- Helpful in patients with subjective, nonspecific complaints; eg, fatigue, dizziness

- Important in ruling out other disease, such as mass lesions in posterior fossa, craniocervical junction, or cervical cord

*Prognosis***

- Extent of disease at presentation has significant prognostic value

Disease Activity

- Provides a method to determine if the disease is active when uncertainty exists on clinical grounds

Disease Severity

- Useful in determining severity of disease; eg, amount of T_2 lesion abnormality, and amount of tissue destruction (T_1 holes and atrophy)

*Monitor MS Course****

- Helpful in determining whether a patient's disease is quiescent while on therapy

- Key outcome measure in clinical trials of new therapies

     * See Chapter 3
   ** See Chapter 2
*** See Chapters 8 and 9

Solitary or confluent nodular lesions are near to or contiguous with the lateral ventricles, and are also seen more peripherally in the cerebral white matter. Lesions occur in the subcortical white matter, in the brain stem and cerebellum, and in the cervical and thoracic spinal cord. The fluid-attenuated inversion recovery (FLAIR) sequence is an imaging technique that is heavily T_2-weighted but suppresses the water signal derived from cerebrospinal fluid (CSF). This increases the conspicuousness of T_2 lesions, which are often contiguous with the brain ventricles. This technique may allow more precise quantification of T_2 lesions on standard MRI scans (Figure 4-2).

Only 5% of new brain lesions observed with MRI are clearly related to new neurologic signs, and these lesions are usually located in the spinal cord, optic nerves, or brain stem. The vast majority of new MRI lesions, particularly hemispheric lesions, are 'clinically silent.' Over time, T_2 lesion volume increases by 5% to 10% yearly in patients with relapsing-remitting multiple sclerosis (RRMS), but significant month-to-month fluctuations occur, and the methodology for precise quantification has not been fully standardized. In patients with a clinically isolated syndrome (CIS) or RRMS, the correlation between the number and volume of T_2 lesions and clinical features is weak, but the number and volume of these lesions at the CIS stage predict the risk of conversion to definite MS later on. The amount of increase in T_2 lesion volume during the first 5 years after CIS predicts clinical disability and brain atrophy 14 years later. Consequently, the effect of disease-modifying drug therapy (DMDT) on T_2 lesions during the early stage of MS has been of great interest.

On T_1-weighted images obtained after administration of the paramagnetic agent gadolinium DTPA (GdDTPA), some of the lesions were brightly enhanced (Figure 4-3). Gadolinium-enhanced lesions represent foci of active inflammation. Gadolinium-enhanced lesions arise in previ-

Table 4-2: Brain MRI Abnormalities in Multiple Sclerosis Patients

Type	Appearance
Lesions	
T_2 lesion	Bright (white) on T_2-weighted images
Gadolinium-enhanced lesion	Bright (white) on T_1-weighted images after gadolinium administration
T_1 black hole	Black or gray on T_1-weighted images without gadolinium administration
Whole Brain Changes	
Brain atrophy	Loss of brain parenchymal volume and increased size of ventricles and subarachnoid spaces

ously normal white matter, or within areas of T_2 lesions, persist for 4 to 8 weeks, and then subside. Such lesions come and go with variable frequency, as illustrated in Figure 4-4, but occur with a frequency about 10 times greater than clinical relapses. Their frequency is weakly correlated with disability or brain atrophy over the short term and with future brain atrophy severity.

T_1 hypointense lesions appear black or gray on T_1-weighted images without gadolinium administration (Figure 4-5). They are frequently termed 'black holes.' Black holes are observed transiently in acute lesions (where they represent edema within the lesion), and in more chronic lesions with severe tissue destruction and axonal loss. The

Comments

Increase 5% to 10% per year during RRMS.
Increasing T_2 lesion volume during RRMS correlates
with MS-related disability and brain atrophy in later years.

Indicates active lesion.
Gadolinium-enhanced lesion study is the most common
screening tool for new therapies.

Observed transiently with acute lesions.
Observed in chronic lesions (eg, longer than 6 months
after lesions form).

Occurs early in the course of MS.
Reflects axonal and myelin destruction.

volume of T_1 black holes is 15% of the T_2-lesion volume,
but varies considerably between patients. The volume of
black holes correlates more strongly with clinical disability than does the T_2-lesion volume.

Brain and spinal cord atrophy have been documented
in MS patients using various image-processing methods
(Figure 4-6). Brain volumes begin to deviate from age-
matched normals within a few years of MS onset, and
decline at a fairly steady rate during the course of disease,
though the rate of atrophy varies considerably among patients. In both RRMS and secondary progressive MS
(SPMS), atrophy rates are 5-fold to 10-fold higher than
those of age-matched healthy controls.

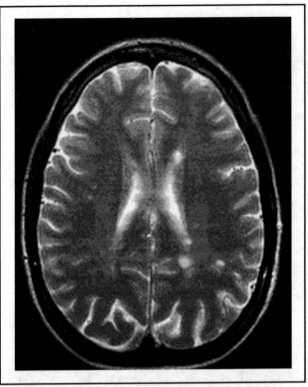

Figure 4-1: T_2 hyperintense lesions on cranial magnetic resonance imaging scan. T_2-weighted axial image through the body of the lateral ventricles, showing two periventricular lesions on the left side, a left-sided lesion in the corpus callosum, and lesions in the parietal white matter.

Diagnosing Multiple Sclerosis

Testing with MRI has been incorporated into making the diagnosis of MS; most MS experts believe that MS should not be diagnosed without it. Brain MRI is abnormal in 95% of patients with definite MS, and lesions are

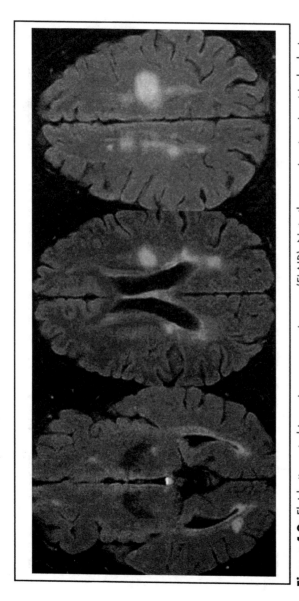

Figure 4-2: Fluid attenuated inversion recovery images (FLAIR). Note the prominent periventricular lesions and clear delineation from the ventricular and subarachnoid cerebrospinal fluid.

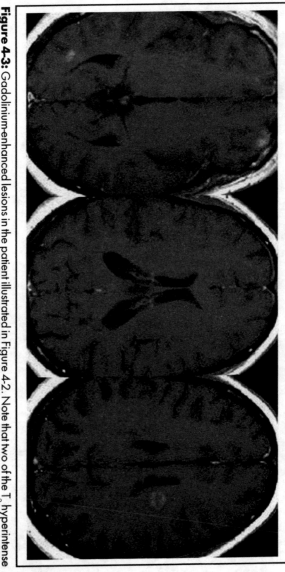

Figure 4-3: Gadolinium-enhanced lesions in the patient illustrated in Figure 4-2. Note that two of the T_2 hyperintense lesions from Figure 4-2 also enhance after gadolinium administration, indicating that the lesions are new or recent.

demonstrable in the spinal cord in more than 70% (Figure 4-7). Complete absence of lesions is strong evidence against a diagnosis of MS. The pattern of lesion distribution is important to diagnosis. Lesion characteristics are listed in Table 4-3.

Such MRI findings are suggestive, but there is no pathognomonic pattern. Diagnosis must be consistent with the clinical features. A common source of confusion is nonspecific small, peripheral white matter lesions related to aging per se in a patient with only nonspecific symptoms, such as fatigue. Because age-related lesions do not occur in the spinal cord, MRI is useful in older patients when results from brain imaging are normal or equivocal.

The McDonald Diagnostic Criteria cited in Chapter 3 incorporate MRI more specifically than any prior diagnostic scheme. According to the McDonald Criteria, MS can be diagnosed in patients presenting with CIS, provided there is MRI evidence for disease dissemination in time and space, as defined in Tables 4-4 and 4-5. Studies demonstrated high specificity and sensitivity for clinically definite MS if at least three of the four criteria in Table 4-4 were present.

Prognosis of Multiple Sclerosis

Follow-up studies have shown that MRI lesions at the time a patient presents with CIS increase the likelihood of clinically definite MS. The longest follow-up study to date (14 years after the initial episode) showed that 88% of patients with an abnormal MRI at presentation had developed clinically definite MS, compared with 19% who had normal baseline MRI scans. Gadolinium-enhanced lesions at the time of presentation, nine or more T_2 lesions at baseline, spinal cord as well as brain lesions at baseline, and a new T_2 lesion 3 months later all significantly increase the likelihood of developing clinically definite MS within the next 2 years.

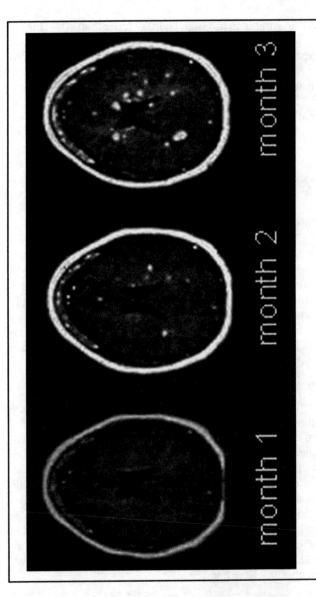

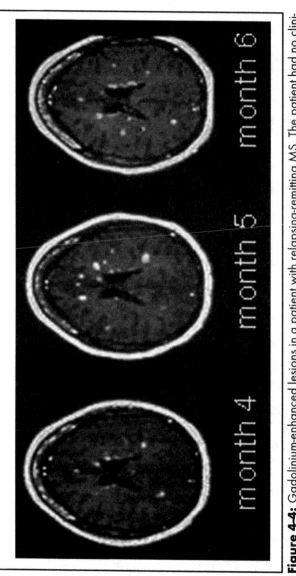

Figure 4-4: Gadolinium-enhanced lesions in a patient with relapsing-remitting MS. The patient had no clinical relapses during the 6-month observation. Note the numerous gadolinium-enhanced lesions in the periventricular white matter. Lesion number varied from month to month.

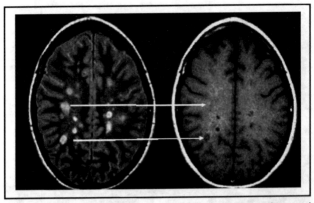

Figure 4-5: T_1 hypointense lesions evident in the right panel (black holes). Some of the T_2 hyperintense lesions evident in the left panel demonstrate black holes on T_1 weighted images (bottom arrow), while many of the T_2 lesions are not accompanied by T_1 black holes (top arrow).

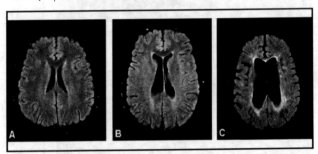

Figure 4-6: Brain atrophy in MS. Cranial MRI scans showing brain atrophy in MS compared with a healthy control. **A.** From a 31-year-old healthy male control. **B.** From a 36-year-old woman with RRMS, 2 years' duration. **C.** From a 43-year-old woman with secondary progressive MS, 19 years' duration.

The study mentioned above, which described patients followed for 14 years from presentation with CIS, helped clarify the role of MRI in predicting disease progression.

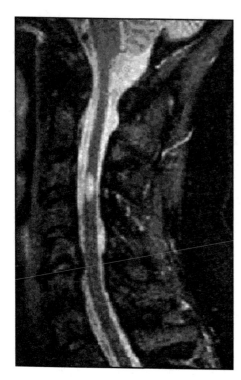

Figure 4-7:
T_2 hyperintense lesion within the cervical spinal cord.

MRI was performed at baseline, and repeated at 5, 10, and 14 years. The median change in T_2 volume during the follow-up was a 10-fold increase. Significant correlations existed between T_2 volumes at early visits and disability at year 14. The strongest correlation with disability at year 14 was with T_2 volume at year 5 and the change in T_2 volume between onset and year 5, indicating that MRI T_2 lesion load and T_2 lesion growth during the early stages of MS predict long-term disability. However, the strength of the prediction was only moderate. Approximately one third of the variability in disability between patients at 14 years' disease duration could be

Table 4-3: Characteristic Distribution and Appearance of Magnetic Resonance Imaging Lesions in Multiple Sclerosis

Lesions are distributed in the periventricular white matter

- Abutting the ventricles
- Round or ovoid appearance
- Asymmetric involvement in hemispheres

Lesions involving the corpus callosum

- Irregular lesions, best observed on midsagittal sections
- Initially, linear involvement along the inner margin of the corpus callosum

Subcortical lesions

- Abutting or following the gray-white junction

Brain-stem lesions

- Along floor of the fourth ventricle
- Abutting the subarachnoid surface

Spinal cord lesions

- Less than one vertebral segment in length
- Partial cross-sectional involvement
- Wedge-shaped and extending to the subarachnoid surface on axial images
- Gadolinium-enhanced lesions

Table 4-4: Magnetic Resonance Imaging Criteria for Dissemination in Space

Three out of four of the following criteria must exist:

1. At least one gadolinium-enhanced lesion or 9 T_2-hyperintense lesions if there is no gadolinium-enhanced lesion

2. At least one infratentorial (brain stem) lesion

3. At least one juxtacortical lesion (at the gray-white junction)

4. At least three periventricular lesions

Table 4-5: Magnetic Resonance Imaging Criteria for Dissemination in Time

- If a first scan is performed > 3 months after the clinical event, a gadolinium-enhanced lesion is sufficient to demonstrate dissemination in time. If there is no enhanced lesion at this time, a new T_2 or gadolinium-enhanced lesion at least 3 months later fulfills the criterion for dissemination in time.

- If the first scan is performed < 3 months after the clinical event, another scan > 3 months after the clinical event showing a new gadolinium-enhanced lesion provides sufficient evidence for dissemination in time. If no enhanced lesion is seen at this second scan, a further scan not less than 3 months after the first that shows a new T_2 lesion or an enhanced lesion will suffice.

predicted by the T_2 lesion parameters during the first 5 years. Unfortunately, in later stages of MS, the predictive value of MRI lesions appears to be weaker.

Newer studies have focused on using markers of diffuse brain pathology, such as brain atrophy, as predictors. It was recently shown that progression of whole brain atrophy using the brain parenchymal fraction during the RRMS stage predicts the risk of ambulatory loss 8 years later. Research studies using newer methods for quantifying diffuse brain pathology in early stages of MS are of great current interest.

Monitoring Multiple Sclerosis Therapy

Testing with MRI has been applied to most clinical trials of new DMDT (see Chapters 8 and 9). Gadolinium-enhanced lesions and T_2 lesions are now measured routinely as part of the design of virtually all DMDT clinical trials. Effects of drugs on brain atrophy, or newer MRI methods that evaluate diffuse brain pathology or are more pathologically specific, are of intense research interest. No consensus now exists among MS experts about using MRI to monitor individual patients. For practical reasons, this possibility applies to T_2-weighted and gadolinium-enhanced scans to assess the number of active lesions and lesion load. Quantitative image analysis has not been applied in the routine practice setting, and given the limited overall correlations between standard MRI lesion findings and clinical disability, it may be premature to use imaging features as the principal tool in treatment decisions. As a supplement to the clinical features, however, MRI can be helpful in monitoring individual patients. For example, a normal MRI in a patient with subjective relapses might be reassuring and might obviate the need for aggressive treatment. An active scan, showing new T_2 lesions and new gadolinium-enhanced lesions in a patient on treatment suggests that therapy is not fully effective.

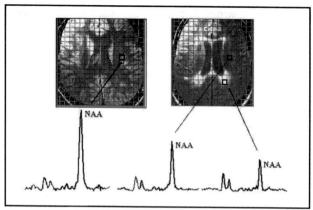

Figure 4-8: Magnetic resonance spectroscopy demonstrating reduced concentrations of NAA. The image on the left is from a healthy control, showing the normal N-acetyl aspartate (NAA) peak (left spectrum). The image on the right is from a multiple sclerosis patient, showing reduced concentrations of NAA in the normal-appearing white matter (middle spectrum), and even lower concentrations in the periventricular lesions (right spectrum). Courtesy of Dr. Doug Arnold, Montreal Neurological Institute.

Magnetic Resonance Measures of Diffuse Brain Pathology

Microscopic pathology is found in macroscopically normal white matter in MS, and quantitative abnormalities in various MRI parameters have been found in the tissue outside the lesions. This appears to indicate a pathologic process that is more diffuse than T_2- or gadolinium-enhanced lesions suggest. The process may include widespread perivascular inflammation, astrocyte hyperplasia, microglial activation, or axonal degeneration at sites distant from macroscopic lesions.

Various techniques have been developed and applied to MS patients. These include magnetization transfer imaging (MTI), which decreases proportionately to the concentration of unbound free water. MTI can be applied to lesions, to nonlesional white matter, and to the whole brain. As tissue integrity decreases, MTI decreases. MTI has been proposed as a method to monitor demyelination, because water molecules within myelin are highly immobile.

Another technique that has gained considerable attention is magnetic resonance spectroscopy (MRS). Of particular interest in MRS studies is a molecule called N-acetyl aspartate (NAA). NAA is restricted to the neuronal/axonal space, and reductions in it have been interpreted as reflecting axonal pathology or loss. Reduced concentrations of NAA have been demonstrated in lesions, and in nonlesion white matter in patients in early stages of MS (Figure 4-8). Thus far, it has proved difficult to standardize the use of MTI or MRS in multicenter studies, so these newer parameters have no current application to individual MS patients in practice settings.

Suggested Readings

Arnold DL, Matthews PM, Francis G, et al: Proton magnetic resonance spectroscopy of human brain in vivo in the evaluation of multiple sclerosis: assessment of the load of disease. *Magn Reson Med* 1990;14:154-159.

Barkhof F, Filippi M, Miller DH, et al: Comparison of MRI criteria at first presentation to predict conversion to clinically definite multiple sclerosis. *Brain* 1997;120(pt 11):2059-2069.

Brex PA, Ciccarelli O, O'Riordan Jl, et al: A longitudinal study of abnormalities on MRI and disability from multiple sclerosis. *N Engl J Med* 2002;346:158-164.

Chard DT, Griffin CM, Parker GJ, et al: Brain atrophy in clinically early relapsing-remitting multiple sclerosis. *Brain* 2002;125 (pt 2):327-337.

De Stefano N, Narayanan S, Matthews PM, et al: In vivo evidence for axonal dysfunction remote from focal cerebral demyelination of the type seen in multiple sclerosis. *Brain* 1999;122(pt 10): 1933-1939.

Filippi M, Dousset V, McFarland HF, et al: Role of magnetic resonance imaging in the diagnosis and monitoring of multiple sclerosis: consensus report of the White Matter Study Group. *J Magn Reson Imaging* 2002;15:499-504.

Harris JO, Frank JA, Patronas N, et al: Serial gadolinium-enhanced magnetic resonance imaging scans in patients with early, relapsing-remitting multiple sclerosis: implications for clinical trials and natural history. *Ann Neurol* 1991;29:548-555.

Kappos L, Moeri D, Radue EW, et al: Predictive value of gadolinium-enhanced magnetic resonance imaging for relapse rate and changes in disability or impairment in multiple sclerosis: a meta-analysis. Gadolinium MRI Meta-analysis Group. *Lancet* 1999; 353:964-969.

Losseff NA, Wang L, Lai HM, et al: Progressive cerebral atrophy in multiple sclerosis. A serial MRI study. *Brain* 1996;119 (pt 6):2009-2019.

Losseff NA, Webb SL, O'Riordan JI, et al: Spinal cord atrophy and disability in multiple sclerosis. A new reproducible and sensitive MRI method with potential to monitor disease progression. *Brain* 1996;119(pt 3):701-708.

McDonald WI, Compston A, Edan G, et al: Recommended diagnostic criteria for multiple sclerosis: guidelines from the International Panel on the diagnosis of multiple sclerosis. *Ann Neurol* 2001;50:121-127.

McFarland HF, Frank JA, Albert PS, et al: Using gadolinium-enhanced magnetic resonance imaging lesions to monitor disease activity in multiple sclerosis. *Ann Neurol* 1992;32:758-766.

Miller DH, Grossman RI, Reingold SC, et al: The role of magnetic resonance techniques in understanding and managing multiple sclerosis. *Brain* 1998;121(pt 1):3-24.

Rudick RA, Fisher E, Lee JC, et al: Use of the brain parenchymal fraction to measure whole brain atrophy in relapsing-remitting MS. Multiple Sclerosis Collaborative Research Group. *Neurology* 1999;53:1698-1704.

Stone LA, Frank JA, Albert PS, et al: The effect of interferon-beta on blood-brain barrier disruptions demonstrated by contrast-enhanced magnetic resonance imaging in relapsing-remitting multiple sclerosis. *Ann Neurol* 1995;37:611-619.

Thorpe JW, Kidd D, Moseley IF, et al: Spinal MRI in patients with suspected multiple sclerosis and negative brain MRI. *Brain* 1996;119(pt 3):709-714.

Truyen L, Van Waesberghe JH, van Walderveen MA, et al: Accumulation of hypointense lesions ('black holes') on T_1 spin-echo MRI correlates with disease progression in multiple sclerosis. *Neurology* 1996;47:1469-1476.

Chapter 5

Pathology and Pathogenesis

Multiple sclerosis (MS) is considered a tissue-specific autoimmune disease that targets the central nervous system. As with other autoimmune diseases, genetic and environmental factors may play a role in susceptibility and severity is extremely variable, even within families. This suggests that disease-modifying genes will be identified that govern disease progression. The concept of MS as an autoimmune disease has led to studies of the mechanism of brain inflammation in MS and of experimental autoimmune encephalomyelitis (EAE) as an informative animal model. MS has not been proven to be an autoimmune disease. In essence, it represents a plausible paradigm of MS etiology, derived from the characteristics of lesion histopathology and from population epidemiology.

Viruses have long been suspected as the underlying cause of MS. Two lines of evidence suggest that viruses can provide a stimulus leading to lymphocyte sensitization against myelin. Patients who develop postinfectious encephalomyelitis after measles virus infection have auto-reactive T cells that recognize myelin protein antigens. Additionally, both naturally occurring viral infection (eg, Theiler's murine encephalomyelitis virus) and experimental viral infection (eg, JHM coronavirus infection of Lewis rats) can produce inflammatory demyelination in rodents. These observations have led to the hypothesis that common viruses may trigger autoimmune demyelination in susceptible patients, leading to the clinical MS phenotype. This is the leading hypothesis for the initial step of the MS disease process—a genetically susceptible individual encounters one of several viral agents capable of generating autoreactive cells during a critical stage of immune-system maturation. After a variable latency, these autoreactive cells become activated, producing clinically apparent disease. As indicated in Chapter 2, there is a well-established link between common viral or bacterial infections and MS relapse. This may result from nonspecific stimulation of pre-existing autoreactive cells. Agents capable of causing relapse, as opposed to initiating the disease, need only provide nonspecific stimulation of autoreactive cells; they do not need to generate them. This concept of MS disease activation was recently supported by the demonstration that nonspecific stimulation with superantigen can generate relapses in the animal model, EAE.

Genetics

From the genetic perspective, MS is considered among the complex diseases of humankind. In a simple genetic disease, disease-causing alleles from a single gene occur rarely in the population, but have a strong effect in leading to the disease. On the other hand, multiple genes contribute a cumulative effect in complex diseases. The genes may be rare or common in the population. In MS, four independent population screens have identified more than 12 common regions of interest within the genome. From the different studies, there are MS-susceptibility regions on chromosomes 5, 6, 17, and 19. Further work is needed to better identify the susceptibility genes, but it is already clear that the genetic basis for MS will be both complex and heterogeneous.

Numerous epidemiologic factors lead to the inevitable conclusion that genetic factors contribute to MS (Table 5-1). There is widely variable prevalence among differing ethnic populations. For example, MS is particularly common in individuals of Northern European descent, but distinctly rare in Asians, American blacks, and Hungar-

Table 5-1: Evidence That MS Is a Genetic Disease

Widely variable incidence/prevalence in different ethnic groups

- Common in people of Northern European descent
- Less common in Asians, Native Americans, Gypsies
- First-degree relatives have a 20-fold to 30-fold increased risk of MS
- Monozygotic twins have a 500-fold increased risk of MS
- Dizygotic twins have the same risk as siblings
- Adoptees and spouses have the same risk as unrelated individuals

ian Gypsies. Family studies have shown that first-degree relatives of MS patients are at least 20-fold more likely to develop MS than unrelated individuals in the same environment, and MS-affected sibling pairs tend to cluster by age of onset rather than year of onset. Genetically unrelated relatives of MS patients, such as adoptees or spouses, are no more likely to develop MS than the population at large, indicating that familial clustering for MS is genetic rather than environmental. Studies of twins pairs showed monozygotic twins have an MS concordance rate of about 50%, a 500-fold increase compared with unrelated individuals in the same environment.

Equally important, 50% of monozygotic twins are discordant for MS, meaning that half of monozygotic twins of an MS patient will not develop MS. This indicates the presence of environmental influence, and implies the interaction between genes and environment.

The most consistent genetic effect identified to date relates to genes encoded in the class II region of the major histocompatibility complex (MHC). The HLA-DR2 haplotype (DRB1*1501 DQB1*0602) located on the short arm of chromosome 6 has been consistently shown to increase risk of MS. MHC class I and II molecules are expressed on antigen-presenting cells. These molecules are responsible for binding and presenting antigenic peptides to CD4+ and CD8+ T cells, which are then activated by a second stimulus to generate an immune response. Binding of peptides to MHC molecules is determined by mutual affinities based on structural characteristics of the MHC molecule and the peptide antigen. Therefore, the simplest interpretation of the MHC-disease association is that polymorphic HLA-DR molecules found in MS patients are more efficient at binding and presenting pathogenic determinants of myelin protein antigens (MBP, PLP, MOG) than are MHC molecules unrelated to MS. Furthermore, it is clear that sequences related to myelin protein epitopes can be derived from the protein components of common viral and bacterial pathogens and can activate myelin-specific T cells. Therefore, the relationship between MHC and MS could be determined in part by the affinity of the HLA-DR2 molecule for these 'molecular mimics' derived from viral or bacterial elements, but interpreted by the host immune system as components of myelin. There is some experimental support for the notion that HLA-DR2 haplotypes associated with MS are 'promiscuous' binders of immune determinants potentially related to disease.

An important research area related to MS genetics is identifying genes that modify the severity or course of MS—so-called disease modifying genes. The HLA-DR2 haplotype associated with increased risk of MS may also convey more rapidly progressive disease, though this has not been totally established. Non-HLA region genes have been associated with more severe MS (eg, the APOE-4 allele), or more mild MS (eg, a variant of the CCR5 gene).

A major challenge in the MS genetics field is to integrate epidemiologic research focused on environmental exposures with whole genome techniques that can define environmental and genetic factors, and elucidate their interaction. The current understanding is that multiple weakly-acting genes interact epistatically with each other, and with environmental factors to determine MS risk in the individual.

Pathology

MS is characterized by lesions disseminated in white and grey matter and varying in age, as would be expected from the clinical features. Because gray matter contains less myelin, lesions in the gray matter are not evident on gross inspection. Consequently, most emphasis until recently has been on white matter lesions, which stand out from surrounding white matter. Figure 5-1 (see color insert) shows the gross pathology in a coronal brain section from a patient dying of MS. In this patient, the lateral ventricles are enlarged as a result of bilateral tissue loss, and there are confluent periventricular plaques. Because of the demyelination, they appear dark brown.

Figure 5-2 (see color insert) shows a microscopic section demonstrating demyelination in an MS plaque. The tissue was stained for myelin stain, which is absent within the lesion.

Lesions occurring separately in the nervous system are in different stages of activity or maturity, implying an evolving process affecting different regions at differing times. The acute lesion is characterized by active inflammatory infiltrates and macrophages containing lipid and myelin degradation products. The chronic, inactive plaque is characterized by demyelination, variable loss of axonal density, glial scar, and absence of inflammation.

Figure 5-3 (see color insert) shows an acute plaque. This lesion has a predilection for periventricular white matter, but may be scattered throughout the CNS. The acute plaque begins with margination and diapedesis of lymphocytes and macrophages forming perivascular cuffs about capillaries and venules. This is followed by diffuse parenchymal infiltration by inflammatory cells, edema, astrocytic hyperplasia, myelin stripping from axons by macrophages and microglia, increased numbers of lipid-laden macrophages, and demyelinated, dystrophic, or transected axons. As plaques enlarge and coalesce, the initial perivenular distribution of the lesions becomes less apparent. The inflammatory reaction is much less apparent in lesions affecting the gray matter, for unclear reasons. In gray matter lesions, the most prominent pathologic features are diffuse microglial activation, loss of myelin, and neuronal pathology.

Within acute lesions, both myelin and axons are damaged, as illustrated in Figure 5-4 (see color insert). In the figure, three axons are visualized within an acute lesion. Myelin, shown in red in the figure, is damaged along all three axons. One of the axons is transected, and the end of the axon is swollen. The extent of axonal transection in demyelinated areas is variable, but relates to the intensity of inflammation. Over time, with recurrent foci of acute inflammation, cumulative axonal loss from long tracts can be substantial.

Table 5-2 demonstrates the relationship between axonal transection and inflammation. Within active lesions, there are more than 11,000 transected axons per mm^3. In chronic active lesions, there are more than 3,000 transected axons per mm^3 at the leading edge of the plaque where active inflammation and demyelination are evident. Far fewer transected axons are seen in the cellular core of these lesions, and even fewer in the nonlesion white matter near the lesions. These data clearly link inflammation to axonal transection, and suggest that anti-inflammatory strategies would have neuroprotective effects in MS patients.

Inflammatory cells in the acutely demyelinating central area of active plaques stain positive for MHC Class II molecules (DR+). These DR+ cells are mostly microglia and

Table 5-2: Number of Transected Axons in MS Lesions

Activity of the lesions	Transected axons/ mm³ (mean)
Active	11,236
Chronic active	
Edge	3,138
Central core	875
Nonlesion white matter	15
Healthy control white matter	0.7

macrophages, with relatively few T cells and B cells. T cells in the acute plaque are a mixture of CD4+ and CD8+ lymphocytes, which are more numerous near the center of the plaque diminishing peripherally. As a lesion enlarges, T cells become relatively more numerous peripherally, while macrophages take their place centrally. CD4+ cells invade the normal-appearing white matter about the lesion, while CD8+ cells are largely confined to the plaque margins and perivascular cuffs. The plaque margins contain increased numbers of oligodendrocytes, astrocytes, and inflammatory cells. As the lesions become more mature, myelin remnants and macrophages progressively disappear from the central part of the plaque, which eventually becomes a gliotic scar. At the plaque margin, a hypercellular 'glial wall' contains lymphocytes, oligodendrocytes, and a few macrophages and astrocytes. In many instances, the disease process continues with low-grade activity at the plaque margins, manifested by lipid-laden macrophages and lymphocytes, often accompanied by a few thin perivascular cuffs.

Chronic inactive MS plaques have sharply demarcated borders with little hypercellularity. Occasional CD4+ and DR+ cells are scattered through the lesions. A few CD4+,

CD8+, and DR+ macrophages, microglia, and B lymphocytes occur at the edges and also in small numbers throughout otherwise normal-appearing white matter (Figure 5-5; see color insert).

A different pattern of demyelination is less dramatic but more common. It consists of diffusely scattered demyelination involving individual fibers or small groups of fibers interspersed with normal-appearing myelinated fibers. This type of demyelination is accompanied by much more limited, diffuse inflammatory infiltrates.

Plaque-like areas of pale myelin staining, termed 'shadow plaques,' occur in many cases. Shadow plaques have increased cellularity and abnormally thin myelin sheaths of relatively uniform thickness, bearing no relationship to axonal fiber diameter, as in normally myelinated tissue. MS experts believe these shadow plaques represent partial remyelination. This concept is supported by the presence of an increased number of oligodendrocytes–thin myelin sheaths of relatively uniform thickness and short internodal length. It is not clear why remyelination in the shadow plaques is incomplete. In later stages of MS, remyelination is almost completely ineffective. This may occur because of inadequate numbers of oligodendroglia or oligodendroglial progenitor cells, or because of axonal pathology. The latter is suggested by recent findings that large numbers of premyelinating oligodendrocytes are present in chronic MS lesions, but fail to myelinate, as shown in the artist rendition in Figure 5-6 (see color insert). The figure shows a normal oligodendrocyte with normally myelinated CNS internodes (top panel), and an oligodendrocyte observed in a typical chronic MS lesion. The premyelinating oligodendrocytes send out processes that contact axons, but fail to wrap around the axon or to form compact myelin. The cause of this failed remyelination is thought to reside with the axon, which seems incapable of supporting normal myelin formation. An alternative explanation is that there are some inhibitory factors that limit effective remyelination.

Despite a number of reports of 'virus-like particles' seen by electron microscopy of MS biopsy and postmortem material, credible morphologic evidence for the presence of true virions has not been reported. Using newer molecular techniques virus genetic material has been found in MS plaques, but the effort to tie a particular virus to the etiology or pathogenesis of MS has failed so far. Continuing interest focuses on herpesviruses, members of which are neurotropic and characterized by persistence in neurons in latent form with periodic reactivation.

Immunopathology and Lesion Pathogenesis

Infiltration of CNS tissue by circulating leukocytes is thought to be central to MS pathogenesis. Extravasation is mediated by soluble chemoattractants and by mutual pairs of adhesion receptors and counter-receptors on leukocytes and endothelial cells. The adhesion molecules that appear important for entry of cells into MS tissues are the VLA-4 and LFA-1 integrins on leukocytes, which interact with VCAM and ICAM on CNS endothelium. ICAM has been shown to be strikingly upregulated on MS vessels. Chemokines are potent, target-specific chemoattractants that act selectively toward monocytes, T cells, and neutrophils. Both adhesion molecule and chemokine antagonists represent attractive therapeutic strategies for limiting or inhibiting migration of activated hematogenous cells into CNS.

Histopathologically, the MS lesion resembles a delayed type hypersensitivity (DTH) reaction, observed most clearly as a response to intracellular bacteria. CD4+ T lymphocytes and CD8+ T lymphocytes, as well as their cytokine products, have been identified in perivascular infiltrates. Cytokines generated by T cells during DTH reactions are strongly proinflammatory, particularly IFN-γ and TNF-α/β. T-helper 1 (Th1) lymphocytes are T cells specialized to drive DTH reactions. These cells secrete IFN-γ and TNF-α/β, in distinction to T-helper 2 (Th2) cells, which secrete IL-4, IL-5, and IL-10. Th2 cytokines promote antibody responses. Importantly, the cytokine products that drive each limb of the immune response are counter-regulatory towards T cells of the complementary limb. Thus, IFN-γ inhibits Th2 T cells, while IL-4 restrains activation of Th1 cells. For Th1 immune reactions, IL-4 and IL-10 are in effect immunosuppressive. Virtually all known Th1 and Th2 cytokines have been demonstrated in MS lesions. The concept that the Th1 response is pathogenic was strongly bolstered by the observation that treatment with IFN-γ precipitated relapses in MS patients. Despite great interest in the Th1/Th2 hypothesis, it has not been possible to clearly delineate the kinetics of the cytokine response in the MS brain, nor has it been feasible thus far to develop Th2 based cytokine therapy.

There has also been great interest in macrophages and microglia in MS lesions. Traditionally thought to play a passive 'scavenger' role, macrophages appear to be the active effector cells in myelin injury. Macrophages have been observed by electron microscopy to strip and phagocytose intact myelin in a process that may be receptor-mediated. IgG and myelin proteins distributed in a polar distribution on the surface of macrophages in the MS brain suggests that antibodies to myelin may mediate the process of macrophage/microglia-mediated myelin phagocytosis.

In addition to T cells and macrophage/microglia, there is also research interest in B cell activation. There is such significant intrathecal immunoglobulin synthesis in MS patients, that cerebrospinal fluid (CSF) testing for oligoclonal bands or increased IgG has become a diagnostic hallmark (Chapter 3). Selective increase in CSF IgG is evident in 90% of patients with definite MS, and selective increase of IgM or IgA is also observed, somewhat less frequently. The actual role of antibodies in MS tissue injury remains uncertain because no single 'MS antigen' has been identified through immunologic studies of immunoglobulin. Several possibilities might explain the humoral immune response in the MS brain. A brain constituent might stimulate antibodies; the brain protein could serve as a 'target' antigen in a manner similar to the acetylcholine receptor in myasthenia gravis. Alternatively, antigens outside the CNS might stimulate antibodies, but the antibodies might cross-react with normal brain constituents. Finally, a virus might be present in the MS brain but not in the brains of normal individuals. The viral antigens might stimulate antibodies. Extensive studies of immunoglobulin reactivity by many different research groups have led to the conclusion that there is no single antigen to which immunoglobulins are directed. Antiviral antibodies are not the major components of total IgG present in CSF, or the major constituents of oligoclonal bands. However, low titers of IgG antibodies reactive with multiple neurotropic viruses have been repeatedly observed. A similar situation exists for antibrain antibodies in MS. Low concentrations of antibodies have been demonstrated that react with myelin proteins, oligodendroglia, glycolipids, and nuclear antigens.

IgG and complement components have been detected in MS lesions. Tissue-fixed immunoglobulins may activate complement, leading directly to membrane injury, or may result in binding of immune effector cells. Complement activation by tissue-fixed IgG may lead to complexes of late complement proteins (eg, the membrane attack complex), which may in turn mediate myelin injury. Complement activation may also generate fragments of early components such as C3b, which may bind to myelin. Membrane-bound C3b may then bind leukocytes, which mediate tissue injury. Myelin from CNS also activates complement directly, although this has not been shown to occur in vivo. In tissue culture, myelin-mediated complement activation was shown to generate the membrane attack complex and cause membrane injury. This process occurred even in the absence of antibody. Complement components have been measured in CSF from MS patients, and their concentration appears to be altered, indicating complement synthesis in the case of increased concentrations, or consumption in the case of low concentrations.

Recently, MS investigators have begun classifying MS lesions into different categories of immunopathology. Table 5-3 shows a recent classification scheme based on these studies. The most common patterns show T cell-mediated inflammation, either without (pattern 1) or with (pattern 2) evidence of complement activation. Together, these two patterns accounted for about 65% of MS lesions. The third pattern accounts for most of the other cases; it suggests primary pathology in the oligodendrocyte, with limited inflammation and less predilection for blood vessels. So far, lesions in brains from individual patients show only one pattern of MS pathology, suggesting that their different pathologic patterns cause MS in different patients. This would explain why patients respond differently to the same therapy.

Pathophysiology

Figure 5-7 (see color insert) shows two outcomes from inflammation. Axonal conduction failure is an inevitable consequence of inflammation and demyelination. If conduction failure affects the majority of axons in a pathway, patients will experience symptoms (eg, visual loss, weakness, etc). Active inflammation will be clinically silent when demyelination affects a minority of fibers in a pathway. Conduction fails during inflammatory demyelination because of demyelination, and because of damage to sodium channels at nodes of Ranvier. Normally, sodium channels are not present along the axon between nodes (the internodal membrane), so conduction is not possible along the acutely demyelinated axon. Also, membranes at the Nodes of Ranvier are damaged by lysolipids generated by enzymes, particularly phospholipase, present in inflammatory exudates. Phospholipase destroys sodium

channels. Finally, inflammatory mediators such as cytokines or reactive oxygen species inhibit nerve conduction. As inflammation subsides, additional sodium channels are inserted into the axonal membrane, which is a prerequisite for the restoration of nerve conduction along a demyelinated fiber. As this process ensues, conduction is restored and symptoms improve. If damage to the axon is limited, remyelination occurs, though the resulting myelin internodes are shorter and thinner than normal.

Another more serious outcome from inflammation is axonal transection, shown diagrammatically in the second panel of Figure 5-7 (see color insert, and micrograph in Figure 5-4). The mechanism of axonal transection is not known, but it seems likely that the demyelinated axon is vulnerable to the inflammatory environment, and that products of the inflammatory response cause transection. If there are enough viable axons in a pathway, recovery will ensue, and the process of axonal transection will remain clinically silent. Once the process has damaged enough axons, compensatory mechanisms will fail and neurologic function will decline.

Even when conduction is restored in remyelinated fibers, it is not optimal. Fibers that have been remyelinated show temperature sensitivity such that a rise in temperature of as little as 0.5ºC above normal will cause conduction failure in some fibers. The increased influx of sodium that occurs as a result of increased number of nodes and sodium channels at the plaque margin is another important factor. Demyelinated fibers have a poor ability to conduct trains of impulses, in part due to an increased refractory period in the demyelinated segment. In addition, studies in experimentally demyelinated fibers have demonstrated a progressive reduction in longitudinal current amplitude followed by conduction block, which may be because of increased intracellular sodium. The capacity of the sodium pump is soon saturated by increased sodium influx. These features of demyelinated and partially remyelinated fibers relate to motor fatigability and activity-related failure of neurologic function, which are prominent clinically in MS. Also, in an attempt to remove sodium from the axon, activation of the sodium calcium exchanger leads to increased intracellular calcium concentrations. This may be an important pathogenic mechanism of axonal degeneration that complicates the later stages of MS.

Relationship Between Pathogenesis and Clinical Features of MS

In recent years, concepts of MS pathogenesis have evolved rapidly. While MS is still considered an immune-initiated inflammatory disease, there has been increasing awareness of several pathologic features of the disease that have clinical implications: (1) There is expanding recognition that the pathologic process in MS is largely subclinical in its early stages; in many patients, the pathologic process is continuously active despite few symptoms; (2) Axonal and neuronal pathology is much more common than initially thought; axonal pathology is present early during the course of MS, but may be clinically silent during the early stages of the disease; (3) Patients enter the SPMS stage of the disease at a relatively late stage of the pathologic process, probably because the extent of axonal pathology exceeds a threshold.

Traditionally, patients with RRMS have been viewed as having a relatively benign form of the disease, probably because of minimal disability between relapses. Multiple lines of evidence have converged to indicate that the pathologic process is active in RRMS patients, however, and data demonstrate that irreversible tissue injury can accumulate without clinical symptoms during RRMS. These data suggest that the pathological process occurring during the RRMS disease stage leads eventually to SPMS in most patients (Table 5-4).

Approximately 50% of RRMS patients have one or more gadolinium-enhancing lesions on a random cranial

Table 5-4: Data Suggest an Active Disease Process During RRMS

Gadolinium-enhancing lesions occur frequently

Gadolinium-enhancing lesions occur in approximately 50% of RRMS patients on random MRI scans; these lesions occur with about 10 times the frequency of clinical relapses.

New MRI techniques show diffuse brain abnormalities

Magnetic resonance spectroscopy (MRS), magnetization transfer imaging (MTI), and high field strength magnetic resonance imaging show diffuse abnormalities in the normal appearing white matter (NAWM).

Pathology studies demonstrate transected axons

Axons are transected in large numbers in active MS lesions. Axonal transection corresponds to sites of active tissue inflammation, regardless of the disease duration.

Brain atrophy occurs in the early stages of MS

Early in the disease, increasing brain atrophy can be measured in a 1-year period.

MRI scan. These lesions are thought to represent active MS lesions. Each new gadolinium-enhancing brain lesion resolves after 4 to 6 weeks, presumably because acute inflammation resolves. As the gadolinium lesion resolves, a residual T2 lesion is left behind. The volume of T2 brain lesions increases by about 10% per year in RRMS patient groups. Clinical correlation studies have found that most gadolinium-enhancing brain lesions in RRMS patients are asymptomatic, and patients have been observed to have frequent new gadolinium-enhancing lesions with no clinical symptoms whatsoever. This has led to the hypothesis that there is an active pathologic process in RRMS, but that individual new lesions result in symptoms only when the lesion happens to affect a large proportion of the fibers within an articulate part of the CNS (eg, optic nerve or motor tracts). MRI pathology correlation studies have documented acute inflammation at the sites of gadolinium enhancement in MS tissue, and the presence of gadolinium-enhancing lesions correlates with CSF pleocytosis. These findings are consistent with the interpretation that gadolinium-enhancing lesions are a marker for active brain inflammation and, as such, a marker for subsequent MRI and clinical disease activity.

Magnetization transfer imaging (MTI) is an MRI technique that provides information on the structure of CNS tissue. Proton molecules associated with myelin are non-mobile. As tissue water increases, proton molecules become more mobile and magnetization transfer decreases. Because normal CNS white matter consists mostly of myelin membranes, MTI has been proposed as a method to monitor myelin loss. MTI has demonstrated abnormalities not only in lesions, but also in NAWM in sites distant from T2 lesions.

Similarly, magnetic resonance spectroscopy (MRS) has shown abnormalities in the NAWM. These data suggest that the pathologic process in MS occurs earlier and is more widespread than is evident using conventional imaging. MRS studies demonstrated reduced levels of N-acetyl aspartate (NAA), a neuronal marker, in brain lesions, and in NAWM from RRMS patients, suggesting that axonal pathology is a consistent and early feature of the MS disease process. In one study, reduced NAA was observed in cerebral cortex adjacent to subcortical white matter lesions in 8 children with MS, with an average age of 15. Recently, studies from a number of groups have shown reduced NAA in normal-appearing white matter. Interestingly, NAA falls most steeply in normal-appearing white matter during the RRMS disease stage. The studies suggest that inflammation or related pathologic mechanisms result in axonal pathology during RRMS, setting the stage for the secondary progressive stage of the disease.

Simon and colleagues measured the diameter of the III ventricle, diameter of the lateral ventricle, area of the corpus callosum in the midsagittal plane, and the brain width in serial MRI scans from placebo patients with RRMS participating in a clinical trial. After one year and again after two years, there were significant increases in ventricular diameter, and corresponding decreases in corpus callosum area and brain width. This was one of the first of many studies indicating brain tissue loss early in the course of MS. A normalized measure of whole brain atrophy, termed the brain parenchymal fraction (BPF), was also applied to patients in the IFN β-1a (Avonex®) clinical trial. The BPF is derived from the cranial MR image set, by dividing the volume of brain parenchymal tissue by the total volume within the brain surface contour. It represents the proportion of volume within the brain surface, that is, tissue rather than CSF. As brain tissue is destroyed by the pathologic process, CSF spaces are secondarily increased, and BPF decreases. Placebo patients in the Avonex® clinical trial were found to have BPF more than 5 standard deviations below the mean of the healthy control group. BPF decreased significantly during each year of observation. More than 70% of the placebo patients had significant decreases in BPF during the 2-year observation. Decreasing BPF occurred in many patients without clinical relapses, and in many patients without worsening EDSS scores, implying the presence of a subclinical pathologic process resulting in brain tissue loss.

In aggregate, these findings support the hypothesis that MS is active in many patients from early in the disease, but that clinical symptoms only loosely reflect its severity. Why do patients with RRMS function reasonably well and appear stable between relapses? This may occur because compensatory mechanisms are adequate to maintain neurologic function during RRMS. Why do patients with secondary progressive MS develop continued neurologic decline years after the disease onset? This may occur because the extent of irreversible tissue injury has progressed beyond a threshold, where compensatory mechanisms are inadequate to maintain neurologic function. The onset of progressive deterioration is typically delayed for 15 or more years after the onset of relapsing-remitting disease. Intermittent clinical relapses during the RRMS disease stage indicate the presence of the underlying disease process but do not accurately reflect its severity. This may be one of the reasons why the relapse frequency does not accurately predict the long-term prognosis. Once a critical threshold is exceeded, irreversible neurologic disability ensues. Beyond that point, any further disease progression results in progressive disability. This model implies that SPMS represents a relatively late stage of the pathology, and that restorative therapy may be unrealistic at this stage of disease. It also implies the need for proactive monitoring and therapy during the relapsing-remitting stage of MS.

Because of these emerging concepts, many MS experts believe that disease-modifying drug therapy (DMDT) should be initiated early in the course of MS, before irreversible disability has occurred. The rationale for early therapy includes: (1) concerns that the immunologic process leading to tissue injury becomes more complex as time passes, and may be more difficult to control with immunosuppressive therapy; (2) increasing awareness that the inflammatory process is active in many RRMS patients during periods of clinical remission; and (3) concern that the inflammatory process results in irreversible axonal injury, which accumulates over time during the relapsing-remitting stage of MS. These considerations imply that DMDT should be started when MS is definitively diagnosed, because the patient is at risk for subsequent disability progression.

Suggested Readings

Bjartmar C, Kidd G, Mork S, et al: Neurological disability correlates with spinal cord axonal loss and reduced N-acetyl aspartate in chronic multiple sclerosis patients. *Ann Neurol* 2000;48:893-901.

Chang A, Tourtellotte WW, Rudick R, et al: Premyelinating oligodendrocytes in chronic lesions of multiple sclerosis. *N Engl J Med* 2002;346:165-173.

Compston A: The genetics of multiple sclerosis. *J Neurovirol* 2000; 6(suppl 2):S5-S9.

Ebers GC, Sadovnick AD, Risch NJ: A genetic basis for familial aggregation in multiple sclerosis. Canadian Collaborative Study Group. *Nature* 1995;377:150-151.

Haines JL, Ter-Minassian M, Bazyk A, et al: A complete genomic screen for multiple sclerosis underscores a role for the major histocompatability complex. The Multiple Sclerosis Genetics Group. *Nat Genet* 1996;13:469-471.

Lucchinetti CF, Bruck W, Rodriguez M, et al: Distinct patterns of multiple sclerosis pathology indicates heterogeneity on pathogenesis. *Brain Pathol* 1996;6:259-274.

Lucchinetti CF, Brueck W, Rodriguez M, et al: Multiple sclerosis: lessons from neuropathology. *Semin Neurol* 1998;18:337-349.

Trapp BD, Peterson J, Ransohoff RM, et al: Axonal transection in the lesions of multiple sclerosis. *N Engl J Med* 1998;338:278-285.

Trapp BD, Ransohoff RM, Fisher E, et al: Neurodegeneration in multiple sclerosis: relationship to neurological disability. *The Neuroscientist* 1999;5:48-57.

Chapter 6

Comprehensive Management of Multiple Sclerosis

P atients with multiple sclerosis (MS) benefit from the expertise of numerous health-care professionals in addition to their physicians. Interactive team-based care, or comprehensive care, is available at many MS centers throughout the world. There is no standard care-team composition; it depends on local expertise and availability of interested professionals. Team members may include the physician (neurologist, urologist, psychiatrist), nurse, physical therapist, occupational therapist, psychologist, social worker, nutritionist, and speech therapist. The nurse often functions as a case manager, providing a central contact with the patient and interface with other team members. The nurse provides education and guidance, manages routine longitudinal care, and directs the patient and family to the other health-care professionals. Rather than fragmenting care, this approach has achieved great popularity. It allows the neurologist to focus on diagnosis (Chapter 3), pharmacologic symptom therapy (Chapter 7), and use of disease-modifying drug therapy (DMDT) to manage the course of the disease (Chapter 8). It also provides a mechanism by which to refer the patient for appropriate rehabilitation and supportive services.

Table 6-1: Key Questions of Newly Diagnosed MS Patients

- What is multiple sclerosis?
- What can I expect will happen to me?
- What will make my illness better, or what will make it worse?
- Can I have children?
- Will my family get MS?

Education and Counseling

Education and counseling are both therapeutic and essential for MS, as they are with other chronic illnesses of uncertain etiology and prognosis. During the early stages of MS, patients are commonly reassured that they have benign MS, or that they look good, but are given insufficient information. They may be told to call if new problems develop, without being told exactly what to look for, and without any focus on their specific questions. Health-care resources are brought to bear on establishing a diagnosis, but little time remains to address questions and concerns of patients, let alone their families. This situation, in turn, can lead to frustration and a breakdown in communication between the patient and the health-care provider.

What follows is a list of commonly encountered questions (Table 6-1) from patients and their families, with suggested answers. This information should be made available to every newly diagnosed MS patient. We have found the answers and explanations to be meaningful and understandable to most patients. The list is not meant to be a complete compendium of necessary information; instead, these responses are offered as a starting point in the education and support process. References and referral sources are listed at the end of the chapter.

Table 6-2: The Process of Inflammation and Demyelination in MS

- *Inflammation:* Invasion of white blood cells, primarily lymphocytes, into the central nervous system. This inflammation causes swelling and damage to surrounding tissue, and may cause neurologic symptoms such as weakness, numbness, or visual blurring. It is responsible for the white spots seen in magnetic resonance imaging (MRI) scans.

- *Demyelination:* Inflammation can lead to damage to the nervous tissue, especially myelin and the underlying axon. Transmission of electrical impulses from one part of the brain to another is more difficult in places where inflammation has occurred. Once the inflammation process has subsided, the nervous system can recover, although the recovery may not be complete. The extent of the symptoms caused by demyelination depends on the location, severity, and duration. If demyelination occurs over an extended time, permanent damage can occur.

- *Axonal loss:* If inflammation is severe enough, the nerve fiber may be severed, resulting in complete loss of electrical conduction, with no recovery.

What is multiple sclerosis?

Patients can better cope with the disease if they can visualize what it is. Table 6-2 provides a factual, simple, but reasonably detailed explanation of the pathologic features of MS, and how they relate to the symptoms the patient is likely to experience. The best evidence indicates that MS (literally translated 'multiple scars') is the result of an autoimmune attack on the central nervous system (CNS), which is made up of the optic nerve, brain, and spinal cord. The attack involves inflammation of the myelin sheath, in a process called inflammatory demyelination. Myelin is the coating that surrounds the nerve fibers, which are also called axons. Myelin serves to protect the axons and to speed nerve conduction. Inflammatory demyelination results in scattered lesions along nerve fibers that damage the myelin and axons, interfering with nerve function. When myelin is stripped away from the axons, electrical impulses are blocked, slowed, or produce irregular signals.

Symptoms in MS patients result from the inflammation process and from damage to the axons. Symptoms vary from one person to another, depending on the location within the nervous system where the inflammation occurs, how widespread the disease is, and how severe or long lasting it has been. Symptoms may resolve completely, or a person may experience some residual effects from an attack. It generally requires 3 months after a relapse to determine how complete the recovery will be.

What can I expect will happen to me?

Life expectancy after MS onset is not changed substantially. Overall, MS patients can expect to live a few years less than the general population without MS, but much of the difference is explained by suicide. Most MS patients develop neurologic disability years after the disease onset. About 20% of patients are unable to walk unassisted or conduct normal work activities 5 years after diagnosis; this percentage increases to 50% by 15 to 20 years, and 75% by 30 years. About 10% to 15% of MS patients experience a benign course, defined as no significant disability after decades of observation.

A hallmark of MS is the unpredictable course of the disease. It is not yet possible at symptom onset to predict whether or when an individual patient will develop disability, or what the future pattern of clinical features will be. Eighty-five percent of patients experience a relapsing-remitting course during the early years of their disease, which is termed relapsing-remitting MS (RRMS). Each relapse, or exacerbation, features a decline in neurologic function developing over a day or two. After about 2 weeks, the patient begins to improve. Recovery is usually substantial or complete during the first 10 years of the disease.

Great variability exists in the recovery time course and eventual outcome following relapses. In many cases no symptoms persist between relapses, particularly in the early years of the disease. The average patient has about one relapse per year, but the pattern is not regular or predictable. After a long interval and following a variable number of relapses, MS commonly changes form. Relapses occur less frequently, are less distinct, and neurologic function begins to decline in a more continuous fashion. Acute relapses may be superimposed on this steady worsening. This stage of the illness is termed secondary progressive MS (SPMS).

It is usually not easy to determine exactly when the RRMS stage ends and the SPMS stage begins because the two disease stages merge over time. SPMS occurs in about 50% of RRMS patients within 15 years after symptom onset. A small proportion of MS patients, probably 15%, develops progressively worse neurologic problems from the beginning, without recoveries and relapses. This is called primary progressive MS (PPMS), and it is not known whether this type of MS has a different cause from the more common RRMS /SPMS variety.

Commonly, PPMS exhibits gradually worsening walking problems because of weakness, stiffness, imbalance, and sensory loss. PPMS usually begins when a patient is in his mid-to-late 40s, as opposed RRMS, which usually begins in the early 30s. There are clinical, magnetic resonance imaging (MRI), and pathologic differences between RRMS/SPMS and PPMS.

Befitting a disease known for its unpredictable nature, MS can exhibit long stable intervals, sometimes decades long, between relapses. The severity of the clinical course of MS during the first 5 to 10 years after symptom onset can be used to roughly predict the eventual course. Favorable prognostic signs during the first 5 years of MS include predominantly sensory involvement with relatively little motor impairment, good recovery from relapses, long intervals between relapses, and mild disease on brain MRI scan. Unfavorable prognostic signs include prominent motor or cerebellar involvement, frequent relapses, poor recovery between relapses, progressive course from onset, and a heavy disease burden on MRI scan. Even with these guidelines, however, precise and accurate predictions cannot be made in an individual patient.

These prognostic markers can be used to make treatment decisions, reserving more aggressive therapy for patients with more worrisome disease characteristics. Patients with favorable characteristics can be reassured and followed by their physicians.

What will make my illness better or worse?

Most patients, or their families, harbor beliefs about the effects of various factors on the MS disease process. These beliefs vary greatly among patients and families, who do not usually express them spontaneously. For example, a mother may believe that her daughter's MS can be controlled by proper nutrition. A wife may believe her husband's stressful job is causing his MS. Sometimes these beliefs are based on misinformation, but more commonly they represent a need to gain some sense of control over the disease. If the patient understands the factors that cause or exacerbate MS, these factors can be controlled. Patients rarely have insight into their need for more control over the disease. Physicians should encourage them to verbalize what they think may improve or worsen their MS. If possible, active control measures should be directed toward healthy behaviors such as proper eating, exercise, stress management, and improved interpersonal relationships. Beliefs that could result in detrimental consequences, such as seeking dangerous or expensive alternative therapies without proven value, should be actively discouraged. Many patients regain a sense of control by learning the facts about MS, instituting a fitness program, improving their diet, reducing their weight, and eliminating negative behaviors such as smoking and alcohol or drug abuse.

According to a survey in our center, more than two thirds of patients believe that stress makes MS worse. We tell patients that the evidence on the stress/MS relationship is inconclusive, but we encourage them to pursue approaches to stress reduction as a general health strategy. Patients remember events just preceding relapses, and commonly assign them a causal relationship to MS onset or relapse. For example, a patient may conclude that a divorce or car accident caused the disease. He or she may not verbalize this conclusion, because many patients know that the physician will not be open to the idea. Similarly, patients commonly believe that inoculations or vaccinations precipitate MS activity, although the evidence indicates that vaccination carries no increased risk. Patients should be encouraged to verbalize their beliefs, and then be educated about the facts.

Studies have established that viral illnesses, usually upper respiratory tract infections, can precipitate relapses. Ordinary viral infections should be treated symptomatically. Urinary tract infections (UTIs) also frequently aggravate MS symptoms or precipitate new relapses. Patients should be informed about this, and UTIs must be treated promptly. For patients who have new symptoms, a UTI should be specifically considered and ruled out. Recurrent UTIs should prompt urologic evaluation, and steps must be taken to minimize the risk.

Most MS patients are heat sensitive. They should be counseled that increased core body temperature from a fever or hot weather can cause MS symptoms to reappear. When providing this information, physicians should also inform patients that there is no evidence that increased body temperature will make the MS disease process worse permanently, and that it is not necessary for MS patients to avoid heat exposure. Most MS patients can tolerate warm or hot showers, a day at the beach, or aerobic exercise. Heat sensitivity becomes more of a problem with more severe disability. In a patient who is severely afflicted, fever can be a major problem.

Can I have children?

Most studies have found that women with MS have normal fertility, normal pregnancies, and normal babies. There is no evidence to suggest that one or more pregnancies accelerate progression of disease, and women with MS who wish to have pregnancies should be encouraged. Numerous studies have shown that pregnant women with MS experienced fewer relapses in the second and third trimesters of pregnancy, but more relapses than usual in the first 6 months postpartum. Women should avoid medications during the pregnancy, including DMDT, which should be discontinued before conception, if possible, and reinstituted postpartum. Management of pregnancy, labor, and delivery should be routine, and there is no medical reason to avoid epidural anesthesia if the woman and her obstetrician prefer to use it. Breastfeeding should be supported if this is the wish of the patient. To avoid exhaustion, breastfeeding mothers can pump their breasts in the evening, so that another family member can bottle feed the infant in the middle of the night.

Will my family get MS?

MS is not contagious, and there is no known risk of passing it to a spouse or relative. The risk of MS in the general population is about 0.1% (1 in 1,000). The lifetime MS risk for a first-degree relative of an MS patient (eg, child or sibling) is about 3% to 5% (30 to 50 in 1,000). Although this is greater than the risk in the general population, it is still a small absolute risk. A fraternal twin of an MS patient has the same risk as a non-twin sibling, but an identical twin to an MS patient has a 50% risk of the disease.

Psychosocial Issues

MS, with its unpredictable course and varied symptoms, is an illness that the entire family must learn to deal with. The uncertainty of the disease course creates its own day-to-day stress for a patient, regardless of the level of impairment. Each family member will approach this disease with his or her own coping technique.

Coping Strategies

Coping strategies reflect an individual's personality and style of interacting with the world. When someone is diagnosed with MS, he or she may experience a variety of emotions: denial, fear, depression, or acceptance. Denial is a normal reaction, particularly at the initial diagnosis. Denial can be detrimental, as when the patient needs to make important decisions about treatment options and symptom management.

Fear accompanies the diagnosis for almost all patients. Fear of the unknown (eg, cause, cure, and triggers) influences how a person copes with the disease. For many people, the greatest fear is losing control over their lives. Changes imposed by a chronic illness may lead to bouts of depression. Most people have feelings of sadness or helplessness, but these feelings lift. Others may experience a deeper sense of depression that can interfere with their daily activities of work and family or social life. At times, it may be helpful for the patient or family with MS to seek professional counseling to help deal with changes and challenges prompted by the disease. Accepting the reality of a chronic illness is not easy. In fact, the diagnosis may never be fully accepted. Eventually, most people make the necessary changes in their lives and find that they are paying less attention to the disease and just living their lives.

Reproductive Issues Related to MS
Gynecologic Issues

Gynecologic care for women with MS does not differ significantly from routine practice, aside from a few exceptions relating to drugs commonly used in the MS population. For a proper decision regarding methods of contraception, the physician should consider concurrent medications. Oral contraceptives may be less effective when used with antibiotics that alter their enterohepatic circulation or with medications that induce hepatic enzymes. Immunosuppression may increase the risk of pelvic infection related to the use of an intrauterine device. Barrier contraception should be considered as an alternative for women with MS when frequent antibiotic therapy or immunosuppressive therapies are needed. For women with occasional antibiotic use, oral contraceptives with 50 g estrogen rather than lower-dose pills should be considered. During antibiotic therapy, another method of birth control should supplement oral contraception.

A second concern is the potential increased risk of cervical dysplasia and neoplasia associated with chronic administration of any immunosuppressive drug, including azathioprine (Imuran®). A woman treated with immunosuppressive medications should have a gynecologic examination, including breast examination and pap smear, yearly at a minimum. Women with a history of genital condylomata are particularly at risk. Physicians must carefully consider gynecologic history, with attention to abnormal pap smears or condylomata, before starting chronic immunosuppression therapy.

Effects of MS on Fertility, Pregnancy, and Delivery

MS does not affect fertility or the course and outcome of pregnancy. The number of pregnancies in women with MS was found to be similar to that in a control group of healthy women, and fertility was found to be unaffected by MS. In a study of 70 pregnancies in women with MS, there was no evidence of a 'fetal lethal factor' associated with MS, although there was an increased rate of elective abortions. In 36 pregnant MS patients reviewed by Sweeney, the only obstetric complications were two cases of mild vomiting. Subsequent studies also found no increase in spontaneous abortion, complications of pregnancy or delivery, fetal malformations, or stillbirths. There was no apparent increase in congenital abnormalities or complications of pregnancy, labor, or delivery in a large prospective study. In general, pregnancy in most MS patients is not considered any riskier than in the healthy population.

Management of Pregnancy and Labor in MS

MS is not associated with increased pregnancy complications. If complications arise, including preterm labor, hypertension, preeclampsia, etc, they can be treated routinely. MS also is not associated with increased risk of congenital malformations or poor fetal outcome.

Labor management typically is routine. There is no evidence that MS patients benefit from shortening the second stage of labor. However, maternal exhaustion and resultant increased weakness may require the use of instruments to assist vaginal delivery. Women with severe motor impairment from MS may not be capable of pushing as effectively, and cesarean section should be considered for them. Otherwise, cesarean section should be used only for the usual obstetric indications.

Analgesia with parenteral narcotics or epidural anesthesia can be used as needed. There are no apparent increased complications from epidural anesthesia in women with MS. Epidural anesthesia also does not appear to increase the risk of postpartum relapse. Spinal anesthesia traditionally has been avoided in MS patients, although there are few data comparing its safety in patients with MS vs the general population.

Routine prophylactic steroid treatment is not necessary in women with MS. Physicians must consider steroid coverage during labor and delivery only in women who have received the equivalent of 20 mg of prednisone or more for more than 2 weeks in the recent past. Various regimens have been used when there is concern about possible adrenal insufficiency. A reasonable course is 100 mg hydrocortisone IM on admission to the labor floor, followed by 100 mg of hydrocortisone IM every 8 hours for 24 hours, or until complications are no longer anticipated.

Breastfeeding

MS does not affect a woman's ability to breastfeed, so women with MS are encouraged to breastfeed if they wish to do so. To avoid exhaustion, a schedule to accommodate a full night's sleep should be achieved by augmenting nursing with formula or with pumped, refrigerated breast milk fed to the infant by a helper. There are suggestive—but not definitive—data that breastfeeding decreases the risk of relapse. Issues concerning the use of medications by nursing mothers are examined below.

Effect of Pregnancy on the Course of MS

Some studies have suggested that pregnancy can precipitate the onset of MS. Tillman reviewed the existing data in 1950 and cast doubt on this. Thompson presented data establishing that pregnancy is not associated with an increased risk of MS onset. Of 178 women with MS, only 10 (6%) experienced the onset of disease manifestations during pregnancy, and pregnancy accounted for 10% to 15% of the total follow-up represented in the sample. Thus, the pregnancy months were associated with an expected, or perhaps a slight, decrease in risk of MS onset as compared to nonpregnancy months. In summary, there is no convincing evidence to support the hypothesis that pregnancy causes MS or is associated with increased risk of onset. In contrast, an increased risk of MS onset in the postpartum period would not be unexpected (see below), though there are no data addressing this point.

Though it does not precipitate MS onset, pregnancy does affect the natural course of MS in a predictable manner. Other putative autoimmune diseases, such as rheumatoid arthritis or autoimmune thyroiditis, improve during gestation and worsen in the postpartum period. Most studies suggest that the gestation months, particularly the second and third trimesters, are associated with decreased MS disease activity, reflected in fewer clinical relapses. The rate of relapse in the first 6 months postpartum, however, is increased. The conclusion from many studies is that pregnancy is relatively protective for women with MS, but that the postpartum period is one of increased disease activity and progression. Numerous investigators have found this pattern. MRI studies during pregnancy have also confirmed diminished MS activity during the second half of pregnancy and a return to prepregnancy levels in the first months postpartum. A recent large, multicenter, prospective study focused on 269 pregnancies in 254 women with predominately relapsing MS. In that cohort, the mean relapse rate was $0.7 + 0.9$ in the year before pregnancy. There was a modest reduction in the first two trimesters, and a dramatic, statistically significant decrease to a $0.2 + 1.0$ relapse rate in the third trimester. The relapse rate increased above the previous baseline to $1.2 + 2.0$ in the first 3 months postpartum, and then returned to the previous rate. The actual risk of relapse for an individual MS patient in the postpartum period is 20% to 40%. The increased risk of relapse in the postpartum period suggests that DMDT should be restarted early in the postpartum period in women with previously active disease.

Research to date does not definitively clarify the effect of pregnancy on the ultimate course of MS or accumulation of disability. Overall, there appears to be no obvious, substantial deleterious effect. The lack of definitive information on this question is not surprising. It is difficult to determine the effect of therapeutic intervention on the course of MS generally, and one must study a large, homogeneous group of MS patients, randomize them to two or more interventions, and follow their course without knowledge of the intervention. Such a design obviously is not possible. Also, observational studies will be affected by selection bias, in that women with minimal or slowly worsening disability are more likely to decide to become pregnant compared to women with more aggressive disease. Consequently, there are no data adequate to answer this question definitively.

Birk et al studied eight women with MS through pregnancy, each examined twice during pregnancy and twice during the 6-month postpartum period. Six of the eight women experienced postpartum relapses, consisting mostly of mild symptom flares. Disability scores increased between 35 weeks' gestation and 6 months postpartum in six of eight women. For the patients as a group, the mean Kurtzke EDSS score increased from 2.4 at 35 weeks' gestation to 3.4 at 6 months postpartum. While the number of patients was small, this degree of worsening does not seem likely to be caused by the natural history of MS. In contrast, Poser reviewed gestational histories of 512 women with MS and concluded that pregnancy was not associated with an increased rate of disease progression. Similarly, Thompson and colleagues found no relationship between the number of pregnancies and the subsequent level of disability. In the large prospective MS study, pregnancy, epidural anesthesia, or breastfeeding had no effect on short-term accumulation of disability. However, follow-up after pregnancy was relatively short in this study—only 12 months. Thus, while pregnancy or the number of pregnancies does not appear to have a dramatic or predictable effect on worsening disease, its exact effect on the ultimate course of MS remains unclear.

Effect of Disability From MS on Ability to Care for the Baby

Women planning to become pregnant must consider their ability to care for the baby. With preexisting severe disability from motor, visual, or cognitive impairment, it may not be realistic to have a child. A more difficult issue is long-term prognosis in women with early, mild disease.

For patients with MS as a group, the median time to moderate impairment is 8 years from the onset of symptoms. The median time from symptoms onset to the need for an assistive device to walk is 15 to 20 years. Because there is substantial heterogeneity in course, it is impossible to predict with certainty the prognosis for individual patients. Unfavorable prognostic signs, as reviewed earlier in this chapter, can be used to guide the patient's decision regarding this issue.

Common Questions About Reproductive Issues
Should I have a baby?

This often is the ultimate question that women with MS contemplating a family face. The decision to have a baby should be based on a range of clinical, personal, family, and economic issues, among which is the presence of MS. Rarely should the decision be based exclusively on the presence of MS. It is recommended that physicians support a couple's decision to have a baby in the face of MS, particularly if physical impairment is not severe and the couple is committed to the plan. The physician should take an educational, supportive, and optimistic role in helping a couple with the decision to have a baby (Table 6-3).

Will pregnancy make my MS worse?

Data suggest that pregnancy is associated with decreased risk of relapse, but there is an increased risk for 6 months postpartum, as reviewed earlier. The risk of postpartum relapse is about two to three times the expected relapse rate. In the individual patient, the risk for a postpartum relapse is probably 20% to 40%. There should be a plan for adequate help in the home to assist with infant care and nighttime feedings. Women with MS should plan to take 3 to 6 months of maternity leave from work, if possible.

Can I decrease the risk of postpartum relapse?

No measures are shown to decrease the risk of postpartum relapse. Adequate rest and alleviation of stress in the postpartum period seem prudent and may diminish the frequency or severity of relapses. Also, DMDT should be restarted or considered after delivery to reduce the risk of relapse.

Will my ultimate disability be worse as a result of pregnancy?

Currently available data suggest that pregnancy does not alter the overall course of MS, including long-term disability. One must exercise caution in rendering an opinion on this question, however, because prior studies are not definitive.

Will MS affect the management of my pregnancy?

Once pregnant, a woman with MS typically requires routine care. She should take prenatal iron to avoid anemia. A high index of suspicion for and prompt treatment of UTIs is vital. Both MS and pregnancy are associated with increased UTIs, and pyelonephritis is a serious complication of pregnancy. Therefore, prophylaxis with nitrofurantoin (Macrodantin®) or ampicillin (Principen®) should be considered for patients with a history of recurrent UTIs or if intermittent catheterization is required.

Will pregnancy affect the management of my MS?

Options for disease-modifying treatment of MS and MS-related symptoms are more limited during pregnancy. Nonessential medications should be avoided during pregnancy.

Will termination of pregnancy affect my disease?

Pregnant MS patients should not terminate their pregnancies because of MS. There appears to be some risk of relapse following termination of pregnancy at any time during gestation. However, there are few data concerning this point.

Will I pass MS on to my children?

There is an increased lifetime risk of MS in the offspring of mothers or fathers with MS, in the range of 2% to 3%. Physicians should inform the patient about this increased risk, stressing that the actual risk of transmission is small.

Management of MS During Pregnancy

Making the Diagnosis of MS During Pregnancy

On occasion, women develop acute CNS syndromes during pregnancy for which the diagnosis of MS is considered. In general, the evaluation for suspected MS can be carried out without concern for the fetus. Cranial MRI is considered safe, but ideally one should wait until after the first trimester. Spinal MRI and gadolinium should be avoided. Lumbar puncture, evoked potentials, and screening blood work for alternative diagnoses can be performed without risk to the fetus.

Pharmacotherapy of MS During Pregnancy

The teratogenic potential of many drugs in humans and the advisability of their use in pregnancy have been established by the US Food and Drug Administration (FDA). Category A drugs have been demonstrated to be safe in humans in trials involving pregnant women. Such data exist for few medications. Category B drugs have data showing no harm to the fetus in animals, but no definitive human data. Cat-

Table 6-4: Medication Therapy During Pregnancy

	Drug	FDA Category
Disease-modifying therapy	Glatiramer acetate	B
	Interferon β-1a	C
	Interferon β-1b	C
	IVI g	C
	Azathioprine	D
	Cyclophosphamide	D
	Cladribine	D
	Methotrexate	X
Acute relapses	Methylprednisolone	C
	Prednisone	C
	ACTH	C
Fatigue	Pemoline	B
	Fluoxetine	B
	Amantadine	C

egory C drugs have been shown to produce harmful effects in animals, but again with no definitive human data. Category D drugs have a demonstrated risk for deleterious effects on the fetus in humans. For Category B, C, and D, the physician should carefully weigh the need relative to the potential risk. Category X drugs carry a known substantial risk to the fetus and are contraindicated in most circumstances. In general, treatment regimens should be reviewed and unnecessary drugs should be eliminated, when possible, before conception. The FDA pregnancy categories for the drugs commonly used in MS are summarized in Table 6-4.

	Drug	**FDA Category**
Spasticity	Baclofen	C
	Tizanidine	C
	Gabapentin	C
	Diazepam	D
Detrusor hyperactivity	Oxybutynin	B
	Propantheline	C
	Tolterodine	C
Pain	Carbamazepine	C
	Gabapentin	C
	Amitriptyline	C
	Nortriptyline	uncertain
	Phenytoin	D

A small number of women have become pregnant while undergoing treatment with interferon β-1b (Betaseron®), interferon β-1a (Avonex®), or glatiramer acetate (Copaxone®) and have had healthy babies. The type I interferons are abortifacient, and both interferon β-1b and β-1a are classified as Category C. Glatiramer acetate is classified as Category B. Nevertheless, there is little information about the safety of these agents during pregnancy. Therefore, it is recommended that women discontinue therapy 1 to 2 months before conception. Therapy can be restarted immediately after delivery and may provide protection against increased risk of relapse in the postpartum period. If a woman becomes pregnant while on interferon or glatiramer acetate therapy, she should stop the medication for the duration of the pregnancy.

Other immunomodulating or immunosuppressive drugs sometimes are used for MS. Intravenous immunoglobulin is not known to be harmful to the fetus in humans (Category C). Azathioprine, cyclophosphamide, and cladribine (Leustatin®) are classified as Category D risks, meaning that there is evidence of fetal risk, but use in selected circumstances may be necessary. Cyclophosphamide is associated with amenorrhea and azoospermia, and carries some risk of permanent sterility. Use of these drugs in pregnancy usually has been associated with a good outcome, but fetal malformations have been reported. For example, a number of pregnancies have been reported in women with systemic lupus erythematosus (SLE) or following renal transplants who took azathioprine, often in association with prednisone. In the largest study, 4 of 44 live-born infants had major congenital anomalies, 23% of the infants were born prematurely, and 24% had low birth weights when born at term. Amniocentesis and fetal ultrasound may assist in assessing fetal development when pregnancy occurs in women treated with these drugs. Methotrexate (Trexall®) is an abortifacient and is contraindicated in pregnancy (Category X).

Corticosteroids are sometimes used to treat MS relapses. They should be avoided if possible, but IV methylprednisolone (Medrol®, Methylpred®) can be used if absolutely necessary for severe relapse. The risk of teratogenicity or virilization of female fetuses is highest in the first trimester, while the risk of fetal adrenal suppression is greatest with high doses of corticosteroids late in gestation. Limited data show no teratogenic effects of adrenocorticotropic hormone (ACTH; Acthar® Gel), but it should be avoided in the first trimester because it may stimulate androgen production and virilization of female fetuses. Studies in rodents show prednisone to be associated with an increased rate of spontaneous abortion, placental insufficiency, and cleft palate. These effects have not been confirmed in humans. Antenatal steroids, commonly betamethasone (Diprolene®, Diprosone®, Lotrisone®), are used to enhance fetal lung maturity when preterm delivery is anticipated and postnatal studies on the infants have shown no adverse effects. Studies in women with various autoimmune diseases, particularly SLE and renal transplant patients, have failed to demonstrate any adverse effects of prednisone, other than neonatal adrenal suppression. In summary, the threshold for treating MS relapses during pregnancy should be somewhat higher than in general practice. Mild relapses may be left untreated. If therapeutic intervention for an acute relapse is absolutely necessary, a short course of IV methylprednisolone is recommended.

Nonessential symptomatic medications should be eliminated before conception and avoided during pregnancy, particularly during the first trimester. A physician should have an increased threshold for symptomatic therapy and treat only intolerable symptoms. When symptomatic therapy is felt to be unavoidable, the safest medication and the lowest dose possible should be chosen. Nonmedication approaches to therapy, when available, should be emphasized.

Light aerobic exercise has been shown to be helpful for fatigue. When medication therapy is deemed to be necessary, pemoline (Cylert®) and fluoxetine (Prozac®, Sarafem®) are the drugs of choice for MS fatigue during pregnancy. Few data exist regarding amantadine (Symmetrel®), although there is one report of two healthy neonates in a woman with MS treated with amantadine throughout the pregnancies. Baclofen (Lioresal®), tizanidine (Zanaflex®), and gabapentin (Neurontin®) all carry some risk to the developing fetus, but can be used if necessary to treat spasticity. Diazepam (Valium®) should be avoided. Oxybutynin

(Ditropan XL®) appears to be the drug of choice for detrusor hyperactivity producing intolerable urinary urgency and frequency. For a bladder that fails to empty, intermittent catheterization should be used. All of the medications used to treat neuropathic pain have been implicated in fetal malformations in humans and particularly should be avoided in the first trimester.

Medication Use by Nursing Mothers

Information about secretion into breast milk does not exist for many of the medications commonly used to treat MS or its symptoms. Because many medications are secreted into breast milk, it is prudent to minimize medication use during nursing. Studies have documented the presence of prednisone in breast milk after doses as small as 5 mg to 10 mg. No studies are available on significantly higher doses analogous to those used to treat MS relapses. Infants have been followed after chronic exposure in mothers taking low doses of steroids and have shown no adverse effects, but few data are available. Renal transplant patients taking azathioprine, known to be excreted in breast milk as 6-mercaptopurine, have breastfed their infants with no apparent adverse effects. We advise against breastfeeding when the mother is using DMDT or immunosuppressive drugs. The use of diazepam by nursing mothers also should be avoided because of infant lethargy, hypoventilation, and weight loss.

Suggested Readings

Birk K, Smeltzer SC, Rudick R: Pregnancy and multiple sclerosis. *Semin Neurol* 1988;8:205-213.

Confavreux C, Hutchinson M, Hours MM, et al: Rate of pregnancy-related relapse in multiple sclerosis. Pregnancy in Multiple Sclerosis Group. *N Engl J Med* 1998;339:285-291.

Damek DM, Shuster EA: Pregnancy and multiple sclerosis. *Mayo Clin Proc* 1997;72:977-989.

Giesser BS: Gender issues in multiple sclerosis. *Neurology* 2002; 8:351-356.

Hartings MF, Pavlou MM, Davis FA: Group counseling of MS patients in a program of comprehensive care. *J Chronic Dis* 1976; 29:65-73.

Lorenzi AR, Ford HL: Multiple sclerosis and pregnancy. *Postgrad Med J* 2002;78:460-464.

McFarland HF, Greenstein J, McFarlin DE, et al: Family and twin studies in multiple sclerosis. *Ann N Y Acad Sci* 1984;436:118-124.

Mueller BA, Zhang J, Critchlow CW: Birth outcomes and need for hospitalization after delivery among women with multiple sclerosis. *Am J Obstet Gynecol* 2002;186:446-452.

Roullet E, Verdier-Taillefer MH, Amarenco P, et al: Pregnancy and multiple sclerosis: a longitudinal study of 125 remittent patients. *J Neurol Neurosurg Psychiatry* 1993;56:1062-1065.

Sadovnick AD, Dircks A, Ebers GC: Genetic counselling in multiple sclerosis: risks to sibs and children of affected individuals. *Clin Genet* 1999;56:118-122.

Smeltzer SC: Reproductive decision making in women with multiple sclerosis. *J Neurosci Nurs* 2002;34:145-157.

Thompson DS, Nelson LM, Burns A, et al: The effects of pregnancy in multiple sclerosis: a retrospective study. *Neurology* 1986; 36:1097-1099.

Voskuhl RR: Gender issues and multiple sclerosis. *Curr Neurol Neurosci Rep* 2002;2:277-286.

Worthington J, Jones R, Crawford M, et al: Pregnancy and multiple sclerosis—a 3-year prospective study. *J Neurol* 1994;241: 228-233.

Chapter 7

Symptom Management of Multiple Sclerosis

Spasticity

Spasticity is a velocity-dependent increase in muscle tone. It is part of the upper motor neuron syndrome, resulting from pathology in the corticospinal tract and the associated descending motor pathways. The syndrome includes loss of dexterity, weakness, hyperactive reflexes, clonus, spasms, and extensor plantar responses. In patients with multiple sclerosis (MS), spasticity predominately affects the legs, but in more advanced cases the patient's trunk and arms are involved. At the mild end of the spectrum, problems may include motor fatigability, loss of dexterity, or difficulty with running and hopping. In more severe cases, patients experience severe stiffness, pain, weakness, and spasms. The spastic gait appears stiff with short steps, at times with scissoring of the legs. Ambulation may acquire a bouncing quality. Spasticity can be detected by a rapid stretch of affected muscle groups, which produces a 'catch' followed by a 'release.' The supine position will unmask leg spasticity. In more severe cases, even slow, passive movement is difficult because of extreme resistance.

Optimally, spasticity should be managed using a comprehensive approach, involving medication and physical therapy. Physicians and therapists should outline the goals of spasticity treatment for the patient—including pain reduction, less frequent or severe spasms, greater mobility, and improved sleep. Complicating factors such as intercurrent illness or infection should be treated independently, although these often occur as spasticity worsens. Proper positioning also reduces spasticity. Simple measures such as flexion at hips and knees during sleep can reduce spasticity significantly.

Antispastic drugs fall into four categories: γ-aminobutyric acid (GABA) agonists, benzodiazepines, skeletal muscle relaxants, and α-2 adrenergic agonists. Baclofen (Lioresal®), the only selective GABA-B agonist available, is a first-line spasticity drug. The therapeutic window is wide and the optimal dose must be individually determined. Treatment usually begins with 5 mg t.i.d., and the patient is instructed to increase the dose by 5-mg to 10-mg increments every 3 days, as needed. Mild cases may respond to doses ranging from 5 mg t.i.d. to 10 mg q.i.d. Moderate spasticity usually requires 10 mg to 20 mg q.i.d. More severe cases may require more than 200 mg per day, if tolerated. The principal limitations of baclofen are increasing weakness, which emerges as muscle tone is reduced, and sedation or confusion. The latter is a particular problem in patients with forebrain disease. Patients should be cautioned against abruptly discontinuing baclofen, which may cause withdrawal seizures.

For severe spasticity, baclofen can by infused into the lumbar subarachnoid space by an implanted infusion pump (intrathecal baclofen [ITB]). Intrathecal baclofen should be considered in patients with severe spasticity complicated by contractures, disruptive spasms, difficult positioning, or pressure sores. The ITB pump is fully implantable in the abdominal subcutaneous space and programmable via an external transmitter. The rate of baclofen can be adjusted easily to achieve optimal therapeutic responses and to minimize toxicity. Complex schedules are possible. For example, baclofen can be administered primarily at night if problems are largely restricted to those hours. The total daily dose of baclofen administered intrathecally is only 1% to 2% of the required oral dose, and ITB usually does not cause sedation or confusion because baclofen distribution is limited to the spinal cord. Treatment with ITB is often effective when oral agents are not, such as in the case of severe spasticity with associated pain and uncontrolled spasms. In severely disabled patients who are nonresponsive to conservative management and oral medications, ITB dramatically reduces spasticity and spasms in more than 90% of cases.

Increasingly, ITB has been used in ambulatory patients with significant spasticity, but this should be restricted to research centers to ensure proper patient selection.

Noradrenergic α-2 agonists act within the spinal cord to enhance noradrenergic-mediated polysynaptic inhibition. In addition to demonstrated effects on spasticity and spasms, these drugs exert antinociceptive effects mediated by α-2 receptors in the dorsal horn of the spinal cord. Tizanidine (Zanaflex®), the only drug of this class approved for the treatment of spasticity in the United States, is also a first-line agent for the treatment of spasticity. Clinical trials of tizanidine demonstrated benefits on spasticity and spasms similar to that of oral baclofen. Tizanidine tends to cause less weakness than baclofen, but this benefit is offset by a high incidence of sedation. Other side effects include dry mouth, dose-dependent hypotension, hepatic transaminase elevations, and rarely, hepatic dysfunction. The usual starting dose is 2 mg at bedtime with gradual escalation of the dose to a maximum of 36 mg per day in 3 to 4 divided doses. Combination therapy with oral baclofen has not been formally tested, but is used routinely in clinical practice.

Gabapentin (Neurontin®), an anticonvulsant used as adjunctive therapy for partial seizures, has been useful for paroxysmal motor and sensory phenomena in patients with MS. Although structurally similar to the inhibitory neurotransmitter GABA, gabapentin does not interact with the GABA receptor and its mechanism of action is unknown. Gabapentin is a useful adjunctive agent for treatment of spasticity, especially nocturnal spasms. For patients who tolerate baclofen or tizanidine poorly, gabapentin can be combined with lower doses of the standard drugs. The initial dose of gabapentin is 100 mg t.i.d., which can be increased gradually to a maximum 900 mg t.i.d. Although tolerated at higher doses, benefit with dose escalation beyond 900-mg t.i.d. is uncommon. For nocturnal spasms, gabapentin can be used as a single bedtime dose. The principal side effect of gabapentin is sedation, usually a problem only during the initial weeks of therapy.

Benzodiazepines, such as diazepam (Valium®) or clonazepam (Klonopin®), are effective drugs for spasticity and spasms, but their use has been largely supplanted by baclofen and tizanidine. Small doses of diazepam (eg, 2 mg t.i.d.) can be used in combination with baclofen for difficult spasticity, and nocturnal spasms can be treated effectively with benzodiazepines, even when spasms do not respond to other drugs. For nocturnal spasms, diazepam, 5 mg to 15 mg q.h.s., or clonazepam, 0.5 mg to 2 mg q.h.s., are generally prescribed. This is usually well tolerated, even in patients with forebrain disease.

Dantrolene (Dantrium®) is an alternative antispastic drug that is restricted to nonambulatory patients because of potential hepatotoxicity and tendency to aggravate muscle weakness. Unlike the drugs examined so far, dantrolene exerts its effect at the level of the skeletal muscle by producing a dose-dependent reduction in myofibril contraction. Dantrolene is started at 25 mg at bedtime, and is gradually increased to a maximum dose of 100 mg q.i.d. As a single bedtime dose, dantrolene is well tolerated and effectively controls nocturnal cramps and spasms in patients unable to obtain relief with the previously mentioned agents. As the dose is increased and spread throughout the day, patients may develop diarrhea, anorexia, and nausea. Because of GI side effects, some patients cannot tolerate effective doses. The incidence of toxic hepatitis increases with doses above 400 mg/day and is more common in women and in patients older than 35 years of age. Transaminase levels should be monitored throughout the course of therapy and dantrolene should be discontinued in patients with alanine transaminase (ALT) levels greater than 2 times the upper limit of normal.

Bladder Dysfunction

Eighty percent of patients with MS suffer from bladder dysfunction. Bladder dysfunction impairs social, vocational, and leisure activities, disrupts sleep and normal sexual activity, and can be complicated by urinary tract infection (UTI), kidney and bladder stone formation, renal disease, and, ultimately, urosepsis. The three common categories of neurogenic bladder dysfunction in patients with MS are: (1) failure to store urine, resulting from a low-capacity bladder; (2) failure to empty urine, resulting from a large-capacity atonic bladder, or failure to relax the urinary sphincter during micturition; and (3) combined failure to store or empty urine, usually because of a low-capacity irritable bladder combined with urinary sphincter dysfunction. The third category is characterized by simultaneous contraction of the bladder detrusor muscle and the external urinary sphincter, resulting in high bladder pressures, failure to empty, and retrograde flow into the ureters. This has been termed detrusor-sphincter dyssynergia (DSD), which is accompanied by a high risk of recurrent infection and upper urinary tract involvement. The three conditions cannot be accurately diagnosed by history alone because patients with all three conditions complain primarily about urinary urgency and frequency, nocturia, and urge incontinence. Similarly, urinary hesitancy and a feeling of incomplete emptying—prototypical symptoms of the high-capacity hypotonic bladder—may also be seen in patients with DSD, or even in some patients with the low-capacity irritable bladder.

Patients with significant symptoms should reduce their intake of caffeinated beverages. However, fluid restriction should be discouraged. Patients should be encouraged to acidify their urine with cranberry juice daily to avoid UTIs. All patients with MS with bladder symptoms should have a urinalysis and a culture, if indicated. UTI should be treated. Patients with more than one UTI should have a urologic evaluation. Prophylactic antibiotics should be avoided as the first approach to recurrent infection.

If symptoms do not clear up after the UTI is treated, or if no infection is found, the postvoid urinary residual volume should be determined by ultrasound or with postvoid urinary catheterization. Table 7-1 outlines a management approach based on this testing. A high postvoid residual volume (eg, greater than 100 mL) can be caused by a hypotonic bladder, DSD, or mechanical outlet obstruction, such as with prostatic hypertrophy. This can be managed empirically with intermittent self-catheterization (ISC) every 6 hours. If this fails to relieve symptoms, or if the patient is reluctant to perform ISC, urologic consultation with urodynamic studies will be necessary.

Nocturia can disrupt sleep, which in turn can aggravate fatigue and depression. It can be treated in some cases by evening fluid restriction, anticholinergics, or ISC at bedtime. If this is ineffective, desmopressin acetate nasal spray (DDAVP®), 0.1 mL to 0.2 mL (10 μg to 20 μg) given at bedtime is usually effective. DDAVP® is well tolerated and rarely results in a significant drop in serum sodium levels.

Bowel Dysfunction

Constipation is common in patients with MS. The etiology is not well understood, but is probably complicated by poor dietary habits, immobility, fluid restriction, and concurrent medications (eg, anticholinergics, calcium channel blockers). Bowel incontinence is rare, but can occur in some patients and is disruptive. It usually takes the form of urge incontinence. Excessive bowel motility with bowel frequency is rare, and is easily treated with an anticholinergic medication (eg, hyoscyamine [Levsin®]). For management of constipation and bowel urgency, add-

Table 7-1: Management of Bladder Dysfunction

	Failure To Store
Void Volume	200 mL-300 mL
PVR	<100 mL
Treatment	(1) Anticholinergics: oxybutynin (Ditropan®) 2.5 mg b.i.d. to 5.0 mg t.i.d.; Ditropan® XL 5 mg to 30 mg q.d.; tolterodine tartrate (Detrol®) 1.0 to 2.0 mg b.i.d.; propantheline 15 mg t.i.d. to 30 mg q.i.d.; hyoscyamine (time release) 0.375 mg b.i.d. to t.i.d.
	(2) Urodynamic testing, if anticholinergics ineffective

*Combined failure to store and empty is a complex management problem that requires urologic and urodynamic testing to guide therapy.
PVR = postvoid residual volume

ing a bulk fiber agent such as psyllium (Metamucil®), and increasing water intake, are generally effective.

Sexual Dysfunction

Sexual dysfunction is common even in mild cases of MS, but does not invariably coexist with bladder or bowel problems. Most patients with MS do not spontaneously report sexual dysfunction, but many will readily report it with gentle direct questioning. Erectile dysfunction is the most common problem in men. Women commonly expe-

Failure To Empty	Combined*
<200 mL	100 mL-300 mL
>300 mL	100 mL-300 mL
(1) ISC 4-6 times/d (2) Add anticholinergic, if above ineffective (3) Urodynamic testing, if both ineffective	(1) α-adrenergic blocker terazosin (Hytrin®) 1 mg q.h.s., combine with ISC if PVR >200 mL; or clonidine 0.05 mg b.i.d. to 0.1 mg b.i.d.**; or imipramine (Tofranil®) 10 mg-25 mg t.i.d. (2) Add anticholinergic, if above ineffective (3) Urodynamic testing, if above ineffective

ISC = intermittent self-catheterization
**May also use clonidine patches (0.1 mg-0.3 mg) applied weekly.

rience decreased libido, decreased perineal sensation, and decreased vaginal lubrication. The problem is often multifactorial. Involvement of the lower spinal cord may contribute to symptoms, but psychological factors such as depression and marital discord, as well as the effects of medications, need to be considered. The treatment of erectile dysfunction in men with MS changed dramatically with the introduction of sildenafil (Viagra®). Few patients with MS have known contraindications for treatment with sildenafil, and most respond to doses of 50 mg to 100 mg taken 1 hour before intercourse. Unfortunately, there are still no medications of proven benefit for sexual dysfunction in female patients with MS. Sexual dysfunction can be addressed effectively in specialty clinics that deal with sexual dysfunction in chronic medical diseases.

Tremor and Ataxia

Cerebellar tremor and ataxia are among the most disabling physical MS symptoms and among the most poorly responsive to drug therapy. Therefore, a rehabilitation program should be considered the primary therapeutic approach, supplemented by drug therapy. An occupational therapist can assess adaptive equipment that would maintain independence and safety, and a physical therapist can assist in gait training. Patients with ataxic gait may need a rollator-type walker for safe ambulation. Many drugs have been advocated as treatment for cerebellar tremor in MS. Clonazepam warrants a trial in patients disabled by intention tremor, but before initiating treatment wrist weights should be tried as a simple approach. If ineffective or only partially effective, clonazepam can be started at a single bedtime dose of 0.5 mg. A morning and afternoon dose is slowly added over 10 to 14 days. Thereafter, the daily dose is increased by 0.5 mg every 5 days, always beginning with the evening dose. The dose is gradually increased to an end point of effective control or unacceptable sedation. Rarely do patients tolerate doses in excess of 6 mg per day. Patients should be cautioned to discontinue clonazepam slowly.

Carefully selected patients may benefit from stereotactic ablation of the ventrolateral thalamic nucleus or implantation of a thalamic stimulator. Ideal candidates for thalamic stimulation or ablation are patients who are stable, have moderate to severe proximal tremor of an upper extremity that limits activities of daily living, and who have preserved strength and sensation in the affected limb. The procedure reduces the amplitude of tremor in the contralateral arm; complications include contralateral weakness and cortical deficits such as contralateral neglect or aphasia. Stereotactic thalamotomy should be done only in neurosurgical centers with demonstrated experience.

Fatigue

MS-specific fatigue is described as a feeling of exhaustion, aggravated with exertion, and often worse late in the day. The pathophysiology is unclear because patients can display significant fatigue in the absence of demonstrable motor dysfunction. Patients should be evaluated for causes that are amenable to specific treatment, including coexisting medical conditions such as thyroid disease or anemia, sleep disorder (including frequent awakening caused by nocturia), depression, and aggravating medications. These factors should be treated first, and supplemented by regular exercise to enhance aerobic capacity and endurance, and by simple measures to conserve energy (Figure 7-1).

If no specific factors can be identified, medications can be instituted. Amantadine (Symmetrel®), 100 mg in the morning and early afternoon, is the commonly prescribed first agent. About 30% of patients respond favorably, with side effects that include irritability. Modafinil (Provigil®), a selective wakefulness agent approved for the treatment of narcolepsy, has shown benefit in MS-related fatigue. The mechanism of action is unclear, but it apparently has far fewer side effects than typical central nervous system (CNS) stimulants. Modafinil is generally prescribed to patients who are not responsive to amantadine. The dose is initiated at 100 mg PO each morning and increased to a maximum of 400 mg PO each morning as needed. The most common side effect is headache. Other CNS stimulants, such as pemoline (Cylert®) or methylphenidate (Ritalin®), have been prescribed for the treatment of MS-related fatigue for many years, despite a lack of controlled trials demonstrating efficacy. These medications are considered an option in patients with MS with severe fatigue that is not responsive to the other drugs.

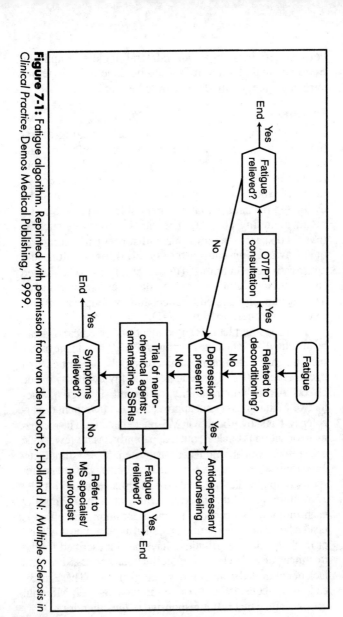

Figure 7-1: Fatigue algorithm. Reprinted with permission from van den Noort S, Holland N: *Multiple Sclerosis in Clinical Practice*, Demos Medical Publishing, 1999.

Heat Sensitivity

MS symptoms frequently worsen or recur in the heat and increased ambient temperature may lead to exhaustion. The etiology is unclear, but it may relate to nerve conduction failure in partially demyelinated axons. Air conditioning during warm months is usually required in the workplace, home, and automobile. If troublesome neurologic symptoms occur because of overheating, cool showers or baths are recommended until the symptom subsides. Fevers associated with infections should be treated promptly with antipyretics and cooling blankets, if needed. Cooling vests have been used by specialized centers and have been shown effective in clinical trials. These can be beneficial in specialized circumstances, such as for patients who are dramatically heat sensitive, or in occupations that do not have air conditioning (eg, factory or construction work).

Pain Syndromes

Pain is common in patients with MS and can be separated into four broad categories: (1) neuralgia; (2) pain from meningeal irritation; (3) centrally mediated dysesthesias; and (4) musculoskeletal pain. An inflammatory lesion in the CNS can affect the dorsal root entry zone of virtually any peripheral or cranial sensory nerve, causing neuralgia. A sharp, lancinating pain may occur spontaneously, or may be triggered by movement or tactile stimulation within the distribution of the affected nerve. Trigeminal neuralgia is a classic example, but glossopharyngeal neuralgia and occipital neuralgia are nearly as common. MS plaques in the cervical spinal cord may produce a pseudoradicular pain, which can be difficult to differentiate from spondylitic radiculopathy. In addition to paroxysmal neuralgic pain, patients with MS may experience constant, severe, aching pain in the same sensory distribution as the neuralgia. At times, this type of pain is more difficult to treat than neuralgia. Treatment of neuralgia begins with gabapentin 100 mg t.i.d., increased as tolerated to a maximum dose of 3,600 mg per day in three or four divided doses. Carbamazepine (Carbatrol®, Tegretol®) is used alone or in combination with gabapentin, beginning at a dose of 100 to 200 mg twice daily. The dose is titrated to pain relief or until unacceptable toxicity occurs. Phenytoin (Dilantin®), amitriptyline, (Elavil®) or baclofen are alternatives to gabapentin or carbamazepine. Patients who do not respond to medications may respond to neurosurgical procedures.

Pain from meningeal irritation occurs during the course of optic neuritis or transverse myelitis, where pain-sensitive dura is stretched or inflamed. Since this typically occurs during acute relapses, pain usually resolves with high-dose intravenous corticosteroids used to treat relapses (see Chapter 8).

Spontaneous dysesthesias, often described as having a burning, prickly quality, are common. Gabapentin, tricyclic antidepressants, or carbamazepine are the most effective drugs for dysesthesias. Doses should be increased gradually to prevent intolerable side effects. Rarely, patients with severe refractory pain may require perphenazine (Etrafon®, Triavil®, Trilafon®) or fluphenazine (Permitil®, Prolixin®) in combination with amitriptyline, although the risk of tardive dyskinesia should be considered.

Musculoskeletal pain is common in patients with abnormal gait and weakness. The lumbar spine, hips, and knees are most commonly affected. Treatment must be directed at the underlying cause. Lumbar back pain in ambulatory patients should be treated with exercise to strengthen the paraspinal and abdominal muscles. Patients too weak to benefit from strengthening exercises may benefit from an elastic lumbar corset. Gait training may improve posture and pain in selected patients. Nonsteroidal anti-inflammatory drugs may relieve pain long enough for patients to participate in physical therapy. Narcotics should be avoided except for short courses to control acute exacerbations of pain. Wheelchair-bound patients with lumbar pain may benefit from a lumbar roll or other types of lumbar support. In many cases, custom cushions for the wheelchair are effective in relieving pain. A custom-fitted ankle-foot orthotic (AFO) device may improve ambulation and pain in patients with foot drop. If a well-fitted AFO fails to relieve knee pain, the addition of a Swedish knee cage or Don Joy brace may further alleviate hyperextension at the knee joint.

Frozen shoulder from chronic tendinitis is common in wheelchair-dependent or bedridden patients with MS. This must be treated aggressively with passive stretching to preserve residual upper extremity function. Intra-articular glucocorticoid combined with an anesthetic may be necessary to allow aggressive physical therapy. Stretching exercises should be continued indefinitely to prevent further recurrences. Hip pain is also common. Avascular necrosis of the femoral heads should be considered in patients receiving frequent pulses of corticosteroids. If hip pain does not respond to conservative management, a magnetic resonance imaging (MRI) scan of the femoral heads may be necessary to evaluate for avascular necrosis.

Patients with MS experience accelerated osteoporosis. Clearly related to immobility from MS, additional risk factors include the postmenopausal state and repetitive pulses of corticosteroids. Patients at high risk should receive prophylactic treatment with calcium supplementation, vitamin D, and hormonal replacement. When appropriate, bone density studies should be obtained to monitor bone density and determine the need for specific osteoporosis treatment. Patients with poorly explained bone pain should be evaluated for fractures related to osteoporosis.

Paroxysmal Motor Symptoms

Paroxysmal motor phenomena are common in MS. The most classic syndrome is the 'tonic spasm.' During a spasm, one arm is forcibly contorted in a dystonic flexion posture.

The ipsilateral leg may be unaffected or may extend forcibly. These spasms last seconds, occur repeatedly, and are painful. Phenytoin and carbamazepine are remarkably effective at controlling these spasms, and may be effective at doses lower than required for seizure control. For minor symptoms without pain, the dose can be increased slowly. Patients unable to tolerate or respond poorly to phenytoin or carbamazepine may respond to gabapentin or baclofen. Treatment is usually continued for 6 months and then the medication is gradually tapered. The spasms do not usually require long-term treatment. Other forms of paroxysmal motor phenomena are less common. Hemifacial spasm, a forceful, grimacing contortion of one side of the face, responds similarly to tonic spasms.

Epileptic seizures occur in 5% of patients with MS, usually late in the course of the disease. A diagnostic evaluation including MRI is necessary to exclude etiologies other than MS. Most commonly, seizures present as a single generalized motor seizure, but focal seizures also occur. Status epilepticus has been reported in MS patients.

Vertigo, Nystagmus, Oscillopsia

Acute vertigo is usually observed in the setting of a brainstem relapse. Treatment consists of intravenous corticosteroids combined with a 1- to 2-week course of a vestibular suppressant. Diazepam at a dose of 2 mg to 5 mg t.i.d. is preferred. Residual vestibular symptoms may respond to vestibular rehabilitation exercises. Chronic ill-defined dizziness is much more difficult to treat. Vestibular testing may be helpful in clarifying the underlying pathophysiology. Alternate diagnoses, such as Meniere's disease, benign positional vertigo, or cerebellopontine angle tumors, are rarely found.

Nystagmus and other oculomotor syndromes may degrade vision and create an illusory motion of the visual environment termed oscillopsia. Pharmacotherapy is generally ineffective, but one trial reported that gabapentin did stabilize images. Some patients may benefit from optical stabilization devices, available at specialized neuro-ophthalmologic centers.

Affective Disorders and Emotional Distress

Emotional distress is common at initial diagnosis, when symptoms recur, and with the development of significant disability that limits usual activities. Clinicians need to maintain a high level of suspicion because patients with MS may not recognize the level of their depression, or even appear depressed. Referral to a psychologist or psychiatrist and use of antidepressants can be helpful to patients. Symptoms such as fatigue, diminished attention and concentration, and pain overlap with MS symptoms. A selective serotonin reuptake inhibitor (SSRI) is generally used as an initial approach to therapy. Commonly used drugs include fluoxetine (Prozac®), sertraline (Zoloft®), paroxetine (Paxil®), or citalopram hydrobromide (Celexa™). For depressed patients with prominent sleep disruption, a small bedtime dose of trazadone (25 mg to 50 mg) can be used together with an SSRI for the first 4 to 8 weeks of therapy. Venlafaxine (Effexor®) is often effective in patients with pain syndromes or decreased libido. For patients with prominent sleep disturbances together with weight loss, tricyclic antidepressants, such as amitriptyline or nortriptyline, may be effective and may be particularly useful if an anticholinergic effect would be helpful for urinary urgency and nocturia.

Bipolar disorder occurs more in patients with MS than in the general population. Treatment is no different from that used to treat bipolar disorders in the general population. Emotional lability, referred to as pathologic laughing and crying, is less common than depression, but disabling. This tends to occur with extensive frontal lobe white matter disease. It is usually controlled with low doses of amitriptyline (ie, 25 mg to 75 mg at bedtime) or with an SSRI.

Cognitive Impairment

MS-related cognitive impairments can be demonstrated in at least 50% of patients, and in some patients may have a devastating impact on activities at school, work, and home. It is important to consider the possibility of cognitive impairment in a patient with MS who is having difficulty with any of his or her roles, if the severity of motor or visual impairment is inadequate to explain the problems. Neuropsychologic testing is required to determine the extent and type of cognitive impairment. Patients with attentional deficits and difficulty concentrating may respond to pemoline, and memory impairment may improve with donepezil (Aricept®).

Suggested Readings

Alusi SH, Worthington J, Glickman S, et al: A study of tremor in multiple sclerosis. *Brain* 2001;124:720-730.

Bagert B, Camplair P, Bourdette D: Cognitive dysfunction in multiple sclerosis: natural history, pathophysiology and management. *CNS Drugs* 2002;16:445-455.

Bakshi R: Fatigue associated with multiple sclerosis: diagnosis, impact and management. *Mult Scler* 2003;9:219-227.

DasGupta R, Fowler CJ: Bladder, bowel and sexual dysfunction in multiple sclerosis: management strategies. *Drugs* 2003;63:153-166.

Krupp LB, Christodoulou C: Fatigue in multiple sclerosis. *Curr Neurol Neurosci Rep* 2001;1:294-298.

Krupp LB, Rizvi SA: Symptomatic therapy for underrecognized manifestations of multiple sclerosis. *Neurology* 2002;58:S32-S39.

Patten SB, Metz LM: Depression in multiple sclerosis. *Psychother Psychosom* 1997;66:286-292.

Rao SM: Neuropsychology of multiple sclerosis. *Curr Opin Neurol* 1995;8:216-220.

Schapiro RT: Pharmacologic options for the management of multiple sclerosis symptoms. *Neurorehabil Neural Repair* 2002;16:223-231.

Taylor A, Taylor RS: Neuropsychologic aspects of multiple sclerosis. *Phys Med Rehabil Clin N Am* 1998;9:643-657.

Chapter **8**

Disease-Modifying Drug Therapy

Chapter 6 covered comprehensive care and education for multiple sclerosis (MS), and Chapter 7 reviewed management of common MS symptoms. This chapter focuses on drug therapy to slow disease progression and improve the long-term outlook for patients with MS. The goals of disease-modifying drug therapy (DMDT) are: (1) to enhance recovery from acute relapse; (2) to reduce the occurrence or lessen the severity of future relapses; and (3) to halt or slow progression of neurologic disability. Treatments that accomplish the second goal—reducing the frequency of relapses—may or may not slow disease progression. Data on this topic vary between clinical trials, and there is controversy in the MS field on the relationship between relapse reduction and the effect on eventual disability progression.

It is important to realize that DMDT is preventive, not restorative. Once neurologic deficits have persisted for 6 months, they tend to be permanent. Therefore, with the exception of acute relapse treatment, DMDT is used to prevent disease worsening. Because of this, DMDT should be considered early in the disease, preferably before a patient has developed significant fixed neurologic deficits. Also, most MS experts agree that MS is more responsive to DMDT at earlier stages, before significant irreversible central nervous system (CNS) injury has occurred and before the patient has entered into the progressive disability stage of the disease. The physician should realize that eventual

Table 8-1: A Typical Protocol for Relapse Treatment With Intravenous Methylprednisolone

Drug	Dose
Intravenous methylprednisolone	1,000 mg q.d.
Oral prednisone	60 mg q.d. 40 mg q.d. 20 mg q.d.
Pepcid®	20 mg q.d.
Mild hypnotic every night as needed	

disease severity cannot be easily predicted early in the illness, so it may be necessary to treat patients with relatively benign disease similarly to patients with more active disease. Hopefully, better predictors of disease severity will emerge to allow more personalized treatment decisions.

Treatment for Patients With a Relapse

Corticotropin and intravenous methylprednisolone (IV MP; Solu-Medrol®) have been documented in controlled trials to hasten recovery from acute relapses. High-dose IV MP may have a more rapid onset of action and may be more effective over time than other steroid preparations. There is some concern about using lower-dose oral steroid preparation for relapses, based on an unexpected finding from the Optic Neuritis Treatment Trial. In that trial, patients with monosymptomatic optic neuritis were ran-

Day	Comment
1-3 (5 days for severe relapses)	Most clinical trial data from studies using methylprednisolone; data exists supporting ACTH gel, other steroid preparations
4-7	Steroid taper may prevent rebound symptoms
8-11	
12-15	
1-15	Prevents gastritis
1-15	Most common side effect is insomnia

ACTH = adrenocorticotropic hormone

domly assigned to placebo; oral prednisone, 1 mg/kg/d; or IV MP at diagnosis. Patients who received IV MP had a much lower relapse recurrence rate compared to placebo patients. Surprisingly, oral prednisone was associated with an increased recurrence rate. This finding has been widely interpreted as suggesting that MS patients who have a relapse and are treated with oral prednisone are at higher risk of 'rebound' relapses; consequently, this has discouraged the use of oral prednisone for MS relapses.

Under what circumstances should patients be treated with IV MP? Current practice is to treat most patients who have relapses accompanied by significant functional impairment. For example, patients with relapses accompanied by visual loss, difficulty walking, and problems with hand dexterity are good candidates for treatment with IV MP. Indiscriminate use of IV MP for symptom fluctuation or for nonspe-

Table 8-2: Disease-Modifying Drugs for RRMS

Drug	Description
IFN β-1a (Avonex®) IFN β-1a (Rebif®)	Recombinant IFN β; glycosylated; amino acid sequence identical with natural IFN β
IFN β-1b (Betaseron®)	Recombinant IFN β; nonglycosylated, cysteine → serine substitution
Glatiramer acetate (Copaxone®)	Random polymer of basic amino acids

RRMS = relapsing-remitting multiple sclerosis
IFN = interferon

cific persistent symptoms such as fatigue should be avoided because there is no class I evidence to support it.

It is common for MS patients to have symptom recurrence during intercurrent viral infection or urinary tract infection. Under these circumstances, observation and treatment of the underlying infection are often adequate.

A commonly used protocol for IV MP therapy is presented in Table 8-1. This treatment can be safely administered in an outpatient setting or in the home by a visiting nurse.

Most patients stabilize or improve within 2 weeks of starting treatment. Neurologic deterioration occasionally occurs during the prednisone taper. In such cases, prednisone can be increased to 60 mg q.d. and tapered more slowly (eg, over 6 weeks). Daily prednisone should not be used over long time intervals.

While this protocol is well tolerated and safely administered in the outpatient setting, patients may require hos-

Possible Mechanisms

Immunomodulatory effects; inhibits cell
migration and cell-mediated inflammation;
? antiviral effects

May regulate T-cell recognition of myelin antigens;
may induce myelin-reactive regulatory cells

pitalization if they have concurrent medical conditions that
require close monitoring during IV MP treatment, such as
diabetes or severe hypertension. Patients may also require
hospitalization for severe relapses that reduce safety at
home (eg, ambulatory patients no longer able to walk).

Common side effects of IV MP include a metallic
taste during the infusion, gastrointestinal upset or ul-
cers, insomnia, flushing, temporary increase in blood
pressure, fluid retention, weight gain, bruising, and hic-
cups. A histamine H_2-receptor blocker (eg, ranitidine
[Zantac®]) or proton pump antagonist (eg, famotidine
[Pepcid®]) can be administered as a single bedtime dose
during the 15 days of steroid treatment. Patients with
insomnia should be given appropriate sedation with a
short-acting hypnotic. Edema should be managed symptomatically with compression stockings and leg elevation rather than with diuretics. On occasion, patients

experience significant depression or hypomania during or after treatment with corticosteroids.

Therapy for Relapsing-Remitting Multiple Sclerosis

Three interferon (IFN) β drugs—recombinant IFN β-1a (Avonex®), recombinant IFN β-1a (Rebif®), and recombinant IFN β-1b (Betaseron®)—are approved for relapsing-remitting multiple sclerosis (RRMS) based on data from phase III clinical trials. Interferon β is a member of the type I IFN family, which includes IFN β and IFN α. Glatiramer acetate (Copaxone®) is also approved for RRMS, based on a phase III clinical trial. Direct comparison of study outcomes for phase III trials of disease-specific therapies for RRMS is difficult because the trials were conducted with similar but not identical study populations, lacked standardized precise outcome measures, and had other differences in design. Tables 8-2 and 8-3 summarize the characteristics and study results of trials of the four drugs approved for RRMS.

Interferon β Clinical Trials

Avonex® and Rebif® are recombinant IFN β preparations that have amino acids identical to those of natural human IFN β. Because the IFN gene product is expressed in a cultured mammalian cell, the molecules are glycosylated like the natural gene product. Betaseron® is produced by *Escherichia coli* cells in culture. It is not glycosylated and substitutes serine for cysteine at the 17 amino acid position.

Interferon β-1b was the first drug approved for RRMS. It was tested in 372 patients who were randomized to placebo, 250 μg (8 million international units [MIU]) IFN β-1b, or 50 μg (1.6 MIU) IFN β-1b by subcutaneous injection every other day for up to 5 years. The primary outcome was a comparison of relapse rates between the three groups. Higher-dose IFN β-1b reduced relapses by 33% and reduced the number of moderate or severe relapses by 50%.

There was a statistically nonsignificant trend suggesting that patients in the 250 µg arm were less likely to experience worsening by at least one point from the baseline Expanded Disability Status Scale (EDSS) lasting for at least 3 months. Interferon β-1b therapy also resulted in a significant reduction in new or enlarging T_2 lesions and reduced the accumulation of T_2 lesion burden shown by magnetic resonance imaging (MRI). The results of this study led to the approval of the 250-µg dose of IFN β-1b to reduce the frequency of relapses in ambulatory RRMS patients.

Avonex® was tested in 301 patients randomized to weekly intramuscular injections (30 µg [6 MIU]) or placebo for up to 2 years. The primary outcome measure was time to onset of sustained disability progression, defined as worsening by at least one point from the baseline EDSS for at least 6 months. Treatment with Avonex® resulted in a 37% lower probability of sustained disability progression, and fewer IFN β-1a recipients became severely disabled, defined as 6-month sustained worsening to at least the EDSS 4.0 or EDSS 6.0 levels. Avonex® also reduced the relapse rate by 32% in the cohort of patients treated for 2 years and by 18% in all patients regardless of the time in the study.

Rebif® was tested in 560 patients who were randomized to receive 44 µg (12 MIU), 22 µg (6 MIU), or placebo by subcutaneous injection three times weekly for 2 years. The primary outcome measure was number of relapses per patient. After 2 years, the lower dose reduced the number of relapses by 29% and the higher dose reduced the number of relapses by 32%. Treatment increased the proportion of relapse-free patients from 16% to 27% in the lower-dose group and from 16% to 32% in the higher-dose group. Rebif® significantly reduced the number of severe relapses, the number of steroid courses, and the number of hospital admissions for MS. There were statistically significant benefits on EDSS change between baseline and 2 years and on the time to 3-month sustained

Table 8-3: Design and Results of Phase III Clinical Trials of Approved Drugs for RRMS

	Avonex®	Rebif®
Sample size for each arm of study	142 (placebo), 158 (30 µg)	187 (placebo), 189 (22 µg), 184 (44 µg)
EDSS	1.0-3.5	0-5.0
Min RR (per year)	0.67 (2 in 3 years)	1.0 (2 in 2 years)
Age (years)	18-55	18-50
Dosage	30 µg (6 MIU) IM weekly	22 µg (6 MIU) SC t.i.w. 44 µg (12 MIU) SC t.i.w.
1° Outcome	Sustained disability	Relapse count
1° Result	Delay in sustained EDSS worsening	29% ↓ (6 MIU) and 32% ↓ (12 MIU)
Adverse events	Flu-like symptoms (first 2-3 months),	Flu-like symptoms (first 2-3 months), skin reactions, increased transaminase

EDSS = Expanded Disability Status Scale, IM = intramuscular, MIU = million international units, RR = relapse rate, RRMS = relapsing-remitting multiple sclerosis, SC = subcutaneous

worsening from the baseline EDSS. These were similar in magnitude to results from the Avonex® study.

Interferon β-1b and IFN β-1a both have beneficial effects on cranial MRI lesions. Betaseron® significantly re-

Betaseron®	Copaxone®
123 (placebo), 125 (50 µg), 124 (250 µg)	126 (placebo), 125 (drug)
0-5.5	0-5.0
1.0 (2 in 2 years)	1.0 (2 in 2 years)
18-50	18-45
250 µg (8 MIU) SC q.o.d.	20 mg SC q.d.
50 µg (1.6 MIU) SC q.o.d.	
Relapse rate	Relapse rate
33% ↓ (8 MIU vs placebo)	29% ↓
Flu-like symptoms (first 2-3 months), skin reactions, increased transaminase	Skin reactions, rare systemic reaction with flushing, sweating, palpitations

duced the number of new or enlarging T_2 lesions in 52 patients studied at one clinical site with MRI scans every 6 weeks, and there was significantly less annual accumulation of T_2 lesions in the entire study group. Betaseron®

also reduced the frequency of gadolinium-enhancing brain lesions. After 1 and 2 years of treatment, Avonex® significantly reduced gadolinium-enhancing brain lesions and decreased the number of new and enlarging T_2 lesions. Rebif® was also found to have prominent beneficial effects on MRI parameters, particularly gadolinium-enhancing lesions and new and enlarging T_2 lesions.

Both IFN β-1a products were tested in patients with clinically isolated syndromes who also had lesions on MRI brain scan. The primary outcome in both studies was to determine if treatment could delay or prevent clinically definite multiple sclerosis (CDMS) in this high-risk population. In the Avonex® study, CDMS developed in 44% fewer IFN-treated patients, and there was a significant reduction in MRI activity in patients who did not develop CDMS. A similar study was conducted with Rebif®, although the dose tested (6 MIU weekly by subcutaneous injection), was lower than that approved for RRMS. Nevertheless, Rebif® significantly reduced the frequency of conversion from clinically isolated syndrome to CDMS.

After the original phase III placebo-controlled clinical trials were completed, many studies were organized to directly compare different products within a single study. The most significant of these studies, the Evidence for Interferon Dose Effect: European-North American Comparative Efficacy (EVIDENCE) trial, compared Avonex® 30 μg (6 MIU) weekly by intramuscular injection with Rebif® 44 μg three times weekly by subcutaneous injection in a randomized, open-label study for 6 months. There were significantly fewer relapse-free Avonex® patients, and the rate of new MRI lesions was higher in the Avonex® patients. In the Rebif® patients, the rate of occurrence of neutralizing antibodies (NAB) was much higher and there were more side effects. The study was designed for a 6-month comparison, but continued follow-up suggested that relapses were similar between the two groups in the next 6 months, suggesting a more rapid onset of clinical benefits with Rebif® compared with Avonex® but similar effects beyond 6 months. Relative efficacy of the two products with longer-term use is unknown

Interferon β Side Effects

The major side effect of IFN therapy is the 'flu-like syndrome.' This usually begins 4 to 8 hours after subcutaneous or intramuscular injection and may persist until the next day. The syndrome includes headache, fever, muscle aches, chills, anorexia, insomnia, lassitude, and fatigue. Flu-like symptoms persist up to 48 hours after each injection. Most patients experience flu-like symptoms when starting treatment. Symptoms persist for more than 3 months in less than 20%. In most cases, symptoms can be managed with acetaminophen or a nonsteroidal anti-inflammatory drug. Some MS experts initiate therapy at half the regular dose, increasing to a full dose over 4 to 12 weeks to lessen flu-like symptoms.

Injection-site reactions occur frequently with IFN products that are administered by subcutaneous injection. They are rare with intramuscular injections. Injection-site reactions consist of swelling, redness, and pain and tend to persist with continued treatment. Approximately 5% of patients develop one or more sites of skin necrosis with subcutaneous IFN. Local injection-site reactions can be managed by applying ice to the injection site or by the use of topical corticosteroids.

Additional side effects include elevated serum transaminase levels, neutropenia, leukopenia, anemia, palpitations, and menstrual irregularities. Hepatic transaminase elevations appear to be more common with the higher-dose IFN products, but they rarely require discontinuation of therapy.

Neurobehavioral side effects, including irritability, anxiety, and depression, are more common with higher-dose IFN products. Depression can be managed with serotonin uptake inhibitors (eg, fluoxetine [Prozac®]) and temporary reduction in dosage. Patients on IFN drugs for MS should be monitored for depression.

Interferon Antibodies

Neutralizing antibodies to IFN occur in about 35% of Betaseron®-treated patients, 25% of Rebif®-treated patients, and 5% of Avonex®-treated patients. The differences are presumed to be related to differences in dose (Avonex® is given in lower doses), physical chemical properties (Betaseron® is nonglycosylated), and routes of administration (Avonex® is given by intramuscular injection; the other products are given subcutaneously). The presence of NAB in the original Betaseron® study was associated with increased relapse and MRI lesion activity, which was similar to patients who received placebo. This observation led to studies to determine the biologic correlates of NAB. Several labs have shown that in the presence of high titers of NAB, the in vivo response to IFN injections is markedly blunted or entirely blocked. Neutralizing antibodies appear between 6 and 12 months after starting therapy. A commercial assay is available to test patient sera for NAB (NAbFeron®). While some MS experts believe that the risk of NAB is a significant issue in selecting an IFN β product and advocate monitoring MS patients receiving IFN drugs for development of NAB, this remains a controversial topic. Not all neurologists agree that NAB are clinically significant, and some neurologists do not monitor patients for NAB.

Glatiramer Acetate Clinical Trials

Glatiramer acetate is a mixture of synthetic polypeptides composed of four amino acids—L-alanine, L-glutamic acid, L-lysine, and L-tyrosine—in a molar ratio of 4.2, 1.4, 3.4, and 1.0, respectively. It was first synthesized at the Weizmann Institute of Science in Israel in 1967. The exact mechanism of action is unknown. Proposed mechanisms in MS include binding to class II major histocompatibility complex with consequent inhibition of myelin-reactive T cells and generation of glatiramer-specific T cells that cross-react with myelin antigens and inhibit the inflammatory response.

Glatiramer acetate was tested in 251 patients given daily subcutaneous injections of 20 mg of the active drug or placebo for 2 years. The primary outcome was the effect of treatment on relapse rate. The original 2-year study reported a 29% reduction in relapse rates in patients treated with glatiramer acetate. Most patients continued in a 1-year blinded extension of the 2-year phase III trial. The reduction in relapse rates was maintained during this additional year of observation.

A European trial was organized after the pivotal phase III study to determine the effect of glatiramer acetate on monthly gadolinium-enhanced MRI scans. Eligibility for this study was restricted to RRMS patients with at least one gadolinium-enhanced lesion on a pre-study MRI scan obtained 1 month before study entry. Patients were randomized to receive glatiramer acetate (20 mg subcutaneously q.d.) or placebo for 9 months, followed by an open-label phase during which all patients received glatiramer acetate. Magnetic resonance images were obtained monthly during the 9-month placebo-controlled phase and then every 3 months for an additional 9 months. The primary outcome—a comparison of the total number of gadolinium-enhanced lesions during the 9-month placebo-controlled phase—demonstrated a 30% to 35% reduction in total enhancing lesions in the patients who initially received glatiramer acetate. Similar reductions were reported for new enhancing lesions and new T_2 lesions. This study demonstrated that the effect of glatiramer acetate on MRI measures of disease activity required 4 to 6 months to develop. Continued observation did not show any further increase in the MRI effect at 18 months. Similarly, a significant reduction in relapse rates did not occur until the last 3 months of the study (months 6 through 9), suggesting that therapeutic effects from glatiramer acetate also required months to develop.

Glatiramer Acetate Side Effects

Glatiramer acetate is generally well tolerated. Mild skin reactions occur in most patients. They can include swelling or tenderness; both are managed with ice and a topical steroid preparation. With prolonged administration, patients may develop focal lipodystrophy at injection sites. The exact incidence of this reaction is unknown. Approximately 15% of patients experience a systemic postinjection reaction that consists of flushing, shortness of breath, palpitations, diaphoresis, and anxiety. The cause of this reaction is also unknown. It can occur early or late in therapy and may recur or be a one-time event. Fortunately, the reaction is self-limited, lasts only minutes, and has never been associated with any significant sequelae. However, patients should be educated about the potential for this reaction to avoid undue panic or concern if it should occur. They should also be informed to seek medical attention if similar symptoms should occur and last more than a few minutes.

Practice Considerations Related to RRMS DMDT

Which is the best interferon preparation?

There is no consensus in the MS field about which of the drug products should be the first-line drug. All three IFN drugs approved for RRMS reduce relapse rate and decrease MRI measures of disease activity. All have favorable long-term tolerability and safety characteristics. Many MS experts think that patients should be treated with the highest possible dose and that the dose of Avonex® is too low. Neurologists with this opinion point to the EVIDENCE study, which demonstrated a benefit of Rebif® compared with Avonex® in reducing relapse rate and new MRI lesions during a 6-month study. Other MS experts believe that the therapeutic benefits of Avonex® compare favorably with the higher-dose products in the different 2-year phase III studies that led to drug approval and point to the significantly reduced risk of NAB and improved tolerability profile for Avonex®.

How does one choose between interferon and glatiramer acetate?

Interferon β and glatiramer acetate are both appropriate first-line agents based on US Food and Drug Administration (FDA) approval for RRMS. Both therapies demonstrated a similar reduction in relapse rates. The MRI effects may favor IFN therapy, particularly if a more rapid onset of therapeutic effect is desired. Multiple studies with IFN β preparations showed a rapid, sustained reduction of more than 70% in new MRI lesions. In contrast, the European Copaxone® study demonstrated a delayed, more modest effect on MRI lesions. There is also more evidence from placebo-controlled clinical trials suggesting a disability benefit with the IFN products. Proponents of Copaxone® point to the risk of NAB with IFN preparations, to the lack of systemic side effects in most patients treated with Copaxone®, and to results from long-term follow-up studies suggesting long-term benefits with Copaxone®.

When should therapy be started?

Studies with the IFN products suggest that early therapy is more effective than delayed therapy. The effects of treatment are largely preventive; the current drugs are useful in preventing new brain lesions and relapses, with the likely benefits of less brain injury and less long-term disability. This implies that therapy should be started as soon as definite MS is diagnosed. Studies at the time of first clinical presentation also provide class I evidence in support of therapy even before a diagnosis of clinically definite MS. Patients with their first clinical episode should be evaluated by a neurologist who is experienced in treating MS patients to consider whether to initiate treatment at that stage.

What is the long-term benefit of early treatment?

Early treatment with DMDT is likely to result in less irreversible brain injury and less long-term disability over time. This has not been demonstrated, however, because the double-blind, placebo-controlled treatment trials are not long enough to determine long-term benefits. Patients in the first Rebif® study were randomized at the end of 2 years to an additional 2 years of controlled follow-up. The

original Rebif® recipients continued on their original dose (22 or 44 µg t.i.w.), and the original placebo patients were randomized to one of the two Rebif® doses. Nearly 80% of the initial study population was followed in this extended study for 4 years. At the end of 4 years, the patients originally treated with Rebif® were less disabled than patients treated with placebo for 2 years followed by Rebif® for 2 years. This study suggests that delaying therapy for 2 years is not desirable. A long-term follow-up study of patients in the first Avonex® study 8 years after the study began also showed that patients who originally received placebo were more disabled than those who originally received Avonex®. In aggregate, these studies suggest that delayed therapy is worse than early therapy, but this point remains controversial because all the evidence is indirect and inferential. Skeptics argue that the cost of the current drugs is not justified by the demonstrated benefits of early therapy. They argue that treatment should be reserved for patients with clearly active disease who are at high risk for converting to secondary-progressive multiple sclerosis (SPMS) and for substantial MS-related disability.

How should patients on DMDT be followed or treated?

MS patients on DMDT should be checked at least yearly for side effects, drug compliance, presence of MS disease activity by clinical and MRI criteria, and various problems requiring comprehensive care or symptomatic therapy, explained in Chapters 6 and 7. In most cases, the patient should receive follow-up care from an experienced neurologist or at an MS center. Disease activity in patients on IFN should prompt testing for IFN NAB. If a high titer of NAB is present, patients should be treated with a less immunogenic IFN product and monitored to determine if NAB disappear or be treated with glatiramer acetate. There are two alternative approaches to NAB-negative patients with continuing disease activity. Neither has been adequately tested in rigorous controlled clinical trials. The first approach involves switching between the monotherapies (eg, from glatiramer acetate to an IFN product or vice versa). The second involves combining drugs with the current drug (eg, adding pulses of methylprednisolone to an IFN product). Studies testing these alternative approaches are now under way.

DMDT for Secondary-Progressive Multiple Sclerosis

Interferon Studies

All three IFN β products were tested in SPMS in double-blind, placebo-controlled studies (Table 8-4). All of the studies enrolled patients who were in the progressive stage of MS and had similar entry disability scores. However, the disease duration differed among the studies, ranging from 13.1 to 16.5 years, suggesting that the studies included different patient populations. All the studies demonstrated beneficial effects on relapse rate and new MRI lesions, but the beneficial effects on measures of disability were mixed. This was especially striking in the IFN β-1b studies. The European Betaferon® study demonstrated a beneficial effect in slowing disability progression measured by EDSS, and this effect was similar in patients with or without pre-study relapses. This result raised considerable optimism in the MS field, because it suggested that IFN treatment was effective in slowing disability even in relatively late stages of the disease. The North American Betaseron® study, using the same drug in a similar patient population, failed to show beneficial effects using the exact same disability outcome measure. This disappointing result is still not well understood. One possibility is that the patients in the North American study were different, and proponents of this argument point to the lower pre-study relapse rate and longer disease duration in the North American study. However, most of the other entry characteristics were similar, and it remains possible that use of the EDSS differed in the two studies.

Randomized trials of Rebif® and Avonex® in SPMS also showed benefits on relapse rate and new MRI lesions, but similar to the North American Betaseron® Study, the results on the EDSS disability measure were negative. The International Multiple Sclerosis Secondary Progressive AVONEX Controlled Trial (IMPACT) used a new disability outcome measure, the Multiple Sclerosis Functional Composite, and demonstrated statistically significant benefits on this scale. The clinical significance of the findings are being debated in the MS field.

The results of IFN β trials in patients with SPMS have thus been mixed, and none of the IFN products has been approved by regulatory agencies for SPMS. The consensus in the MS field is that IFN has at best modest benefits in SPMS patients and that measurable clinical benefits from IFN decline with disease duration. The practical implication is that IFN should be considered in SPMS patients when disease duration is relatively short (eg, less than 15 years) and there is evidence of active inflammation, manifested by new MRI lesions and frequent relapses.

Copaxone® Studies

Two studies of glatiramer acetate were conducted in patients with progressive MS. Unfortunately, both failed to demonstrate clinical benefits. In the first trial, 106 patients with chronic progressive MS were tested for benefits on the EDSS disability scale. There was a trend for less disability progression in the glatiramer acetate group, but it did not reach statistical significance. Another study, the largest trial ever conducted in MS patients, evaluated the effect of glatiramer acetate on disease progression in 943 patients with primary-progressive multiple sclerosis (PPMS). The trial was discontinued early because interim analyses demonstrated no hint of efficacy, and a futility analysis demonstrated that a positive outcome was highly unlikely. Thus, at the present time, there are no data suggesting a therapeutic effect of glatiramer acetate on disease progression in SPMS or PPMS.

Mitoxantrone and Other Immunosuppression Studies

There are no therapies with demonstrated benefits in patients who have advanced SPMS with slow deterioration for years in the absence of relapses or brain inflammation. The early secondary-progressive phase of MS (eg, 10 to 15 years after onset) merges with an early stage of RRMS. Immunosuppressive medications have received the most attention in this setting. Only one drug, mitoxantrone (Novantrone®), has been approved for progressive MS. The specific indication, as cited by the FDA in its approval in October 2000, states that mitoxantrone is approved for "reducing neurologic disability and/or the frequency of clinical relapses in patients with secondary-progressive, progressive-relapsing or worsening relapsing-remitting MS." Mitoxantrone is an anthracenedione, categorized as a chemotherapeutic agent, with potent effects on cellular and humoral immune mechanisms. In clinical trials, mitoxantrone treatment significantly reduced relapse rates, disability progression, and MRI measures of disease activity in active RRMS and SPMS. The major limitation of therapy is dose-dependent cardiac toxicity that limits the duration of therapy to approximately 2 years. Mitoxantrone has also been associated with the development of leukemia in breast cancer patients receiving treatment in combination with radiation therapy and other chemotherapeutic agents, but the risk of leukemia in MS patients receiving mitoxantrone is unclear. Other common adverse effects include nausea, bone marrow suppression, amenorrhea, and infertility. Because of the potential toxicity, mitoxantrone should be prescribed by MS experts with experience in administering chemotherapy or by oncologists experienced in handling this drug.

Smaller phase II studies have suggested that bimonthly pulse therapy with IV MP or low-dose oral methotrexate may slow disability progression in late relapsing MS or early SPMS. Also, several studies have reported benefits from pulse intravenous cyclophosphamide treatment in this phase of the disease. Generally, one of these options may be combined with IFN or glatiramer acetate therapy for patients with evidence of continued disease activity despite monotherapy. However, until randomized, controlled clinical trials are completed, it is not possible to provide evidence-based treatment recommendations for patients entering the SPMS stage despite approved monotherapy with IFN or glatiramer acetate.

Suggested Readings

Beck RW, Cleary PA, Trobe JD, et al: The effect of corticosteroids for acute optic neuritis on the subsequent development of multiple sclerosis. The Optic Neuritis Study Group. *N Engl J Med* 1993;329:1764-1769.

Clanet M, Radue EW, Kappos L, et al: A randomized, double-blind, dose-comparison study of weekly interferon β-1a in relapsing MS. *Neurology* 2002;59:1507-1517.

Cohen JA, Cutter GR, Fischer JS, et al: Benefit of interferon β-1a on MSFC progression in secondary progressive MS. *Neurology* 2002;59:679-687.

Comi G, Filippi M, Wolinsky JS: European/Canadian multicenter, double-blind, randomized, placebo-controlled study of the effects of glatiramer acetate on magnetic resonance imaging—measured disease activity and burden in patients with relapsing multiple sclerosis. European/Canadian Glatiramer Acetate Study Group. *Ann Neurol* 2001;49:290-297.

Goodkin DE, Kinkel RP, Weinstock-Guttman B, et al: A phase II study of i.v. methylprednisolone in secondary-progressive multiple sclerosis. *Neurology* 1998;51:239-245.

Goodkin DE, Rudick RA, VanderBrug Medendorp S, et al: Low-dose (7.5 mg) oral methotrexate reduces the rate of progression in chronic progressive multiple sclerosis. *Ann Neurol* 1995;37:30-40.

Hartung HP, Gonsette R, Konig N, et al: Mitoxantrone in progressive multiple sclerosis: a placebo-controlled, double-blind, randomised, multicentre trial. *Lancet* 2002;360:2018-2025.

Interferon β-1b in the treatment of multiple sclerosis: final outcome of the randomized controlled trial. The IFNB Multiple Sclerosis Study Group, and the University of British Columbia MS/MRI Analysis Group. *Neurology* 1995;45:1277-1285.

Jacobs LD, Beck RW, Simon JH, et al: Intramuscular interferon β-1a therapy initiated during a first demyelinating event in multiple sclerosis. CHAMPS Study Group. *N Engl J Med* 2000;343:898-904.

Jacobs LD, Cookfair DL, Rudick RA, et al: Intramuscular interferon β-1a for disease progression in relapsing multiple sclerosis. The Multiple Sclerosis Collaborative Research Group (MSCRG). *Ann Neurol* 1996;39:285-294.

Johnson KP, Brooks BR, Cohen JA, et al: Copolymer 1 reduces relapse rate and improves disability in relapsing-remitting multiple sclerosis: results of a phase III multicenter, double-blind placebo-controlled trial. The Copolymer 1 Multiple Sclerosis Study Group. *Neurology* 1995;45:1268-1276.

Johnson KP, Brooks BR, Cohen JA, et al: Extended use of glatiramer acetate (Copaxone) is well tolerated and maintains its clinical effect on multiple sclerosis relapse rate and degree of disability. Copolymer 1 Multiple Sclerosis Study Group. *Neurology* 1998;50:701-708.

Neutralizing antibodies during treatment of multiple sclerosis with interferon β-1b: Experience during the first three years. The IFNB Multiple Sclerosis Study Group, and the University of British Columbia MS/MRI Analysis Group. *Neurology* 1996;47:889-894.

Noseworthy JH, Lucchinetti C, Rodriguez M, et al: Multiple sclerosis. *N Engl J Med* 2000;343:938-952.

Panitch H, Goodin DS, Francis G, et al: Randomized, comparative study of interferon β-1a treatment regimens in MS: The EVIDENCE Trial. *Neurology* 2002;59:1496-1506.

Paty DW, Li DK: Interferon β-1b is effective in relapsing-remitting multiple sclerosis. II. MRI analysis results of a multicenter, randomized, double-blind, placebo-controlled trial. UBC MS/MRI Study Group and the IFNB Multiple Sclerosis Study Group. *Neurology* 1993;43:662-667.

Placebo controlled multicentre randomised trial of interferon β-1b in treatment of secondary progressive multiple sclerosis. European Study Group on interferon β-1b in secondary progressive MS. *Lancet* 1998;352:1491-1497.

Randomised double-blind placebo-controlled study of interferon β-1a in relapsing/remitting multiple sclerosis. PRISMS (Prevention of Relapses and Disability by Interferon β-1a Subcutaneously in Multiple Sclerosis) Study Group. *Lancet* 1998;352:1498-1504.

Rudick RA, Goodkin DE, Jacobs LD, et al: Impact of interferon β-1a on neurologic disability in relapsing multiple sclerosis. The Multiple Sclerosis Collaborative Research Group (MSCRG). *Neurology* 1997;49:358-363.

Rudick RA, Simonian NA, Alam JA, et al: Incidence and significance of neutralizing antibodies to interferon β-1a in multiple sclerosis. Multiple Sclerosis Collaborative Research Group (MSCRG). *Neurology* 1998;50:1266-1272.

Simon JH, Jacobs LD, Campion M, et al: Magnetic resonance studies of intramuscular interferon beta-1a for relapsing multiple sclerosis. The Multiple Sclerosis Collaborative Research Group. *Ann Neurol* 1998;43:79-87.

Stone LA, Frank JA, Albert PS, et al: The effect of interferon-β on blood-brain barrier disruptions demonstrated by contrast-enhanced magnetic resonance imaging in relapsing-remitting multiple sclerosis. *Ann Neurol* 1995;37:611-619.

The IFNB Study Group: Interferon β-1b is effective in relapsing-remitting multiple sclerosis. I. Clinical results of a multicenter, randomized, double-blind, placebo-controlled trial. *Neurology* 1993;43:655-661.

Chapter 9

Clinical Trials and Future Approaches to Therapy

Availability of effective drugs for relapsing-remitting multiple sclerosis (RRMS) makes prolonged placebo-controlled trials of unproven therapies ethically questionable. A panel of MS experts concluded that placebo-controlled studies for RRMS are ethical, provided: (1) the patient is informed about the availability of partially effective disease-modifying drug therapy (DMDT); (2) the patient is carefully monitored for disease progression during the trial and offered alternative therapy in the event he or she worsens significantly; (3) there is a strong rationale for the new treatment being tested; and (4) the study is of brief duration. Placebo-controlled studies are considered ethical in progressive MS, regardless of duration, because therapeutic options are much less satisfactory.

In active-arm comparison studies, one active therapy is compared with another, or with active drugs in combination. While common in oncology, active-arm comparison studies have only recently been introduced in MS. The specific designs to conduct such studies in MS are now being developed. Larger sample sizes and more sensitive outcome measures, or both, will be required to show the benefits of new treatments compared with currently available therapies.

Outcome Measures

Table 9-1 lists traditional clinical and magnetic resonance imaging (MRI) outcome measures. Relapse count

Table 9-1: Traditional Outcome Measures for Multiple Sclerosis Clinical Trials

Outcome	Typical Use
Relapses	• Number • Severity • Frequency
EDSS	• Proportion worse by stated amount • Time to worsening by stated amount • Amount of change from baseline
Gadolinium lesions	• Number • Volume
T_2 lesions	• Volume change • Number of new or enlarging lesions

EDSS = Expanded Disability Status Scale

or frequency has been most commonly used, and most neurologists accept relapse as a meaningful outcome measure for MS studies. However, relapses are subjective, and subject to interpretation by both the patient and the neurologist. Symptoms fluctuate from day to day or week to week in many MS patients; it is sometimes difficult to decide whether the problem is symptom fluctuation or relapse. Also, emotional distress and anxiety may drive new symptom reports. Some experts have cautioned against using relapses as an outcome measure in open-label studies, because the relapse rate may be influenced by bias related to patient or physician expectation regarding the effectiveness of test therapies.

Problems

- Relapses are subjective and may be unreliable measures for open-label studies

- EDSS not reproducible
- Most MS patients do not change in 2-year trial
- Numerical change from baseline may not be meaningful because EDSS is an ordinal scale

- Methodology not standardized
- Lesion number depends on dose of gadolinium, technical factors in study
- Not closely linked with disability

- Lesions are pathologically nonspecific
- Methodology not standardized
- Not closely linked with disability

The Kurtzke Expanded Disability Status Scale (EDSS) is also considered a meaningful indicator of MS-related neurologic status and has been used to measure neurologic disability related to MS (Table 9-2). However, it too has many limitations. Studies have shown that different neurologists have difficulty reproducing the same score in the same patient. Because of this difficulty, most studies require the same neurologist to assign EDSS scores to a given patient throughout the course of a clinical trial. This is not always possible for practical reasons. The resulting variability lowers the sensitivity of the clinical trial. Also, studies have shown that patients stay at any given EDSS level for more than 1 year, and for some patients, EDSS average 'staying time' at a given

Table 9-2: Summary of Expanded Disability Status Scale

EDSS 0-3.5	Disability determined by the neurologic examination, as applied to seven functional system scales. Generally, patients in this range have minimal-moderate disability and are able to walk an unlimited distance without assistance.
EDSS 3.5-5.5	Increasing levels of ambulation impairment. Able to walk independently, but ambulation distance is progressively limited.
EDSS 6.0	Requires unilateral assistance (eg, cane) to walk.
EDSS 6.5	Requires bilateral assistance to walk.
EDSS 7.0-9.5	Increasing immobility and need for assistance with activities of daily living.
EDSS 10.0	Dead of MS

level approaches 3 years. Therefore, most patients do not change from one EDSS level to another during the course of a clinical trial, lowering the usefulness of this measure.

Gadolinium-enhanced lesions, or T_2 hyperintense lesions, observed on routine brain MRI studies, are used commonly. New MRI lesions occur frequently, but there is no generally accepted image analysis methodology that would allow precise comparisons from one study to another. Also, gadolinium lesion frequency has not been linked closely with current or future disability, and T_2 lesions are histologically nonspecific. Therefore, T_2 lesion load is only weakly related to disability.

Table 9-3 lists newer outcome measures that have been proposed as more sensitive, reliable, or meaningful. The Multiple Sclerosis Functional Composite (MSFC) was developed by a task force of the National Multiple Sclerosis Society as an improved clinical outcome measure for future clinical trials. It contains three timed tests of neurologic function: a walking test, an arm-dexterity test, and a cognitive test of complex attention. The three test results are normalized using a reference MS population to create a z-score for each test component (representing how close the patient is to the reference population mean performance), and the three z-scores are averaged to create a single score for each patient. The MSFC was found to be highly reproducible when applied by a trained technician to correlate with MRI lesions and brain atrophy, and to change before EDSS changed. The MSFC has already been used in several MS trials, and much more will be learned in the coming years about the value of the MSFC for MS clinical trials.

Brain atrophy has been found to progress slowly in healthy adult controls in the 20- to 55-year age range. However, the rate of brain atrophy was found to be eightfold higher in patients with RRMS. The rapid rate of brain atrophy progression is caused by the pathologic process described in Chapter 5. Brain atrophy measures have been used in MS clinical trials, and they are considered an important component of current MS trials. However, many methods exist for detecting and quantifying brain atrophy, and there is no consensus in the MS field on the optimal method.

One promising approach is based on magnetic resonance spectroscopy (MRS), which uses noninvasive imaging technology to obtain biochemical spectra in brain tissue. It has been possible to identify and quantify spectral peaks; one peak of interest is N-acetyl aspartate (NAA), a neuronal marker. NAA concentrations are reduced in the MS brain early in the disease. Many clinicians hope that MRS methods to quantify NAA will be useful

Table 9-3: Newer Outcome Measures for Multiple Sclerosis Clinical Trials

Outcome	Typical Use
MSFC	• MSFC change from baseline • Slope of MSFC scores over time
T_1 black holes	• Change in volume from baseline • Proportion of new gadolinium lesions that progress to T_1 black holes
Brain atrophy	• Change from baseline
NAA levels by MRS	• Change in concentration relative to choline, a marker peak in the spectra from the MRS study

MSFC = Multiple Sclerosis Functional Composite
NAA = N-acetyl aspartate
MRS = magnetic resonance spectroscopy

for future clinical trials, because the impact of therapies on neuronal number and health is extremely important.

Promising Therapies on the Horizon
Diminishing Autoreactivity to Brain Antigens

Productive interaction between antigen and T lymphocytes requires an MHC class II molecule on the surface of an antigen presenting cell, together with a cognate antigen and T lymphocyte receptor. All three elements contribute to the specificity of the immune response and also to the downstream events resulting from T lymphocyte activation. For example, the nature of costimulatory mol-

Comment

- Was recommended by a National MS Society as an improved clinical outcome measure
- Thought to represent lesions with tissue destruction
- Methodology not standardized

- Very meaningful, relates to destructive pathology
- Methodology not standardized
- Changes very slowly, requiring long studies and large sample sizes

- Most specific method to monitor axonal pathology
- Technically challenging
- Not standardized for multicenter studies

ecules may determine whether a T lymphocyte develops into a memory cell or is immunized to that particular antigen. Work in experimental allergic encephalomyelitis has defined dominant regions of myelin basic protein and defined the therapeutic potential of altered peptides that fail to induce experimental allergic encephalomyelitis and to protect treated animals from active or passive experimental allergic encephalomyelitis induction.

In one study, patients with definite MS were randomized to placebo or CGP77116, an altered peptide based on the amino acid sequence of myelin basic protein 83-99. The study was discontinued because 9% of patients developed hypersensitivity reactions. However, no signs of disease worsening were seen, and one analysis suggested that the volume and number of enhanced lesions were reduced at the highest dose tested (5 mg). In a different study with this altered peptide, several patients had MS relapses, and two also had markedly increased immune reactivity to myelin basic protein. The second study raised a concern about the risk of antigen therapy with this altered peptide.

At present, the future of antigen-specific immunotherapy is uncertain. Treatment with antigen-specific therapies will be complex, because patients vary in myelin recognition patterns and in change over time, and it is not clear how to induce protective as opposed to inflammatory T lymphocyte responses.

Another approach to altering brain tissue autoreactivity is to influence T lymphocyte costimulation. Strategies are being tested based on the signaling systems between T lymphocytes and antigen presenting cells. One such strategy is through a molecule called CTLA4Ig, which may cause autoreactive T lymphocytes to become tolerant. Studies in RRMS are under way.

Strategies to Inhibit Leukocyte Trafficking Into the Brain

Movement of cells across endothelial barriers and into tissue requires numerous molecular events, including interaction between selectins and their integrin receptors on leukocytes; chemokines and their receptors on leukocytes; and enzymes such as metalloproteinases. An attractive therapeutic strategy is to take advantage of the known biology of leukocyte trafficking. This is an active strategy in current clinical trials. Therapy based on blocking chemokine receptors may emerge in the next 5 years.

Inhibiting VLA-4, an a4β1 integrin, has shown promise in early trials and is being tested alone and in combination with other DMDT. A randomized, double-blind, placebo-controlled trial of a humanized monoclonal antibody to VLA-4, natalizumab (Antegren®), was conducted in 213 patients with RRMS or relapsing secondary progressive multiple sclerosis (SPMS). Patients were randomized to 3 mg of intravenous natalizumab per kg (68 patients), 6 mg/kg (74 patients), or placebo (71 patients) every 28 days for 6 months. Natalizumab reduced the mean number of new lesions in both groups: 0.7 in the group given 3 mg/kg natalizumab (P <0.001), and 1.1 in the group given 6 mg/kg natalizumab (P <0.001). The reduction for the placebo group was 9.6 per patient. Twenty-seven patients in the placebo group had relapses, compared with 13 in the group given 3 mg/kg natalizumab and 14 in the group given 6 mg/kg natalizumab.

On the basis of this study, two phase III, randomized, controlled clinical trials are being conducted to determine the benefits and risks of natalizumab. In the first trial, natalizumab is being compared with placebo in RRMS patients. In the second, patients with disease activity despite interferon β-1a (Avonex®, Rebif®) were randomized to added placebo or natalizumab.

More Aggressive, Early Immunosuppression

An important direction in MS therapy is the use of aggressive immune suppression, such as mitoxantrone (Novantrone®), bone marrow transplantation, or anti-CD52 therapy with alemtuzumab (Campath®) early in the disease. This approach is based on the hypothesis that therapy delayed even 5 years after the first symptom may be ineffective, but that the same therapy applied early in the disease might give long-lasting remission, or even cure. Such studies are being considered.

Neuroprotection Strategies

Increasing awareness of axonal degeneration as a mechanism for disability progression has led to studies related to the mechanism of axonal degeneration. These studies have provided new insights and potential strategies to protect axons. An important factor in future MS therapeutic strategies will be to add drugs that protect axons.

Complementary and Alternative Medicine

The MS field has witnessed many therapeutic claims, ranging from snake venom through bee stings. Generally, these claims are unsubstantiated. However, with the emergence of complementary and alternative medicine as a rigorous therapeutic discipline, many therapies are being tested. These include mind-body therapies such as relaxation, imagery, or reiki; dietary therapy based on hypothesized effects of nutrition; and food additives. Thus far, none of these approaches has been shown to change the natural course of the disease, but many trials are planned and some are ongoing.

Suggested Readings

Conlon P, Steinman L: Altered peptide ligands and MS treatment. *Science* 2002;296:1801-1802.

Cutter GR, Baier ML, Rudick RA, et al: Development of a multiple sclerosis functional composite as a clinical trial outcome measure. *Brain* 1999;122 (Pt 5):871-882.

Filippi M, Horsfield MA, Ader HJ, et al: Guidelines for using quantitative measures of brain magnetic resonance imaging abnormalities in monitoring the treatment of multiple sclerosis. *Ann Neurol* 1998;43:499-506.

Kalkers NF, Bergers L, de GV, et al: Concurrent validity of the MS Functional Composite using MRI as a biological disease marker. *Neurology* 2001;56:215-219.

Kappos L, Moeri D, Radue EW, et al: Predictive value of gadolinium-enhanced magnetic resonance imaging for relapse rate and changes in disability or impairment in multiple sclerosis: a meta-analysis. Gadolinium MRI Meta-analysis Group. *Lancet* 1999; 353: 964-969.

Lublin FD, Reingold SC: Placebo-controlled clinical trials in multiple sclerosis: ethical considerations. National Multiple Sclerosis Society (USA) Task Force on Placebo-Controlled Clinical Trials in MS. *Ann Neurol* 2001;49:677-681.

Martin R, Bielekova B, Gran B, et al: Lessons from studies of antigen-specific T cell responses in multiple sclerosis. *J Neural Transm Suppl* 2000;361-373.

McFarland HF, Barkhof F, Antel J, et al: The role of MRI as a surrogate outcome measure in multiple sclerosis. *Mult Scler* 2002;8:40-51.

Miller DH, Barkhof F, Frank JA, et al: Measurement of atrophy in multiple sclerosis: pathological basis, methodological aspects and clinical relevance. *Brain* 2002;125:1676-1695.

Miller DH, Khan OA, Sheremata WA, et al: A controlled trial of natalizumab for relapsing multiple sclerosis. *N Engl J Med* 2003; 348:15-23.

Miller DM, Rudick RA, Cutter G, et al: Clinical significance of the multiple sclerosis functional composite: relationship to patient-reported quality of life. *Arch Neurol* 2000;57:1319-1324.

Noseworthy JH: Multiple sclerosis clinical trials: old and new challenges. *Semin Neurol* 1998;18:377-388.

Petkau J: Statistical methods for evaluating multiple sclerosis therapies. *Semin Neurol* 1998;18:351-375.

Rovaris M, Filippi M: Interventions for the prevention of brain atrophy in multiple sclerosis: current status. *CNS Drugs* 2003;17:563-575.

Rudick RA, Cutter G, Reingold S: The multiple sclerosis functional composite: a new clinical outcome measure for multiple sclerosis trials. *Mult Scler* 2002;8:359-365.

Sormani MP, Bruzzi P, Comi G, et al: MRI metrics as surrogate markers for clinical relapse rate in relapsing-remitting MS patients. *Neurology* 2002;58:417-421.

Tuohy VK, Yu M, Weinstock-Guttman B, et al: Diversity and plasticity of self recognition during the development of multiple sclerosis. *J Clin Invest* 1997;99:1682-1690.

Wiendl H, Kieseier BC: Disease-modifying therapies in multiple sclerosis: an update on recent and ongoing trials and future strategies. *Expert Opin Investig Drugs* 2003;12:689-712.

Chapter **10**

Internet Resources

People with multiple sclerosis (MS) seek out information about the disease. By obtaining accurate, up-to-date, and objective information, people with MS benefit from a renewed sense of control and well-being. Also, becoming more knowledgeable about MS and its treatment allows more informed decisions and improved collaboration with health-care professionals.

Many sources of information are available, but information is increasingly provided through the Internet. However, the amount of information is so extensive that MS patients, family members, and professionals may be overwhelmed. Also, many Internet sources provide inaccurate or self-serving information.

Therefore, the following list of recommended MS Web sites is provided. Some of these sites provide links to other Web sites that may be of interest.

Multiple Sclerosis Organizations
- **National Multiple Sclerosis Society**—nationally known, nonprofit organization that provides accurate information on MS, current research in MS, and educational programs related to the disease.
  www.nationalmssociety.org
- **The Multiple Sclerosis Society of Canada**—provides information on MS and research.
  www.mssoc.ca
- **World of Multiple Sclerosis/Multiple Sclerosis International Federation**—a comprehensive international

resource developed by MS experts worldwide. Information is available in English, French, Spanish, and German.

www.msif.org

Multiple Sclerosis Resources

- **Cleveland Clinic Health Information Center**—provides information on many health conditions, sponsored by the Cleveland Clinic.
  www.clevelandclinic.org/info
- **InteliHealth**—provides information on a wide variety of health issues, sponsored by Aetna Inc.
  www.intelihealth.com
- **Mayo Clinic Patient Education**—provides information on various health issues, sponsored by the Mayo Clinic.
  www.mayoclinic.com
- **Medscape**—provides information on various health topics.
  www.medscape.com
- **Myelin Project**—international organization dedicated to research on myelin repair.
  www.myelin.org
- **National Library of Medicine**—large medical library on health information, services, and more.
  www.nlm.nih.gov
- **National Center for Complementary and Alternative Medicine**—provides information to the public and professionals on complementary and alternative medicine, supported by the National Institutes of Health.
  www.nccam.nih.gov
- **Quackwatch**—an organization dedicated to fighting health-related fraud. Offers critiques of complementary and alternative medicine.
  www.quackwatch.com
- **Rocky Mountain MS Center**—provides information on the use of current complementary and alternative medicine.
  www.ms-cam.org

- **WebMD**—provides information on a wide variety of health issues, including MS.
  www.webmd.com

Professional Organizations

- **American Academy of Neurology**—provides resources for medical professionals.
  www.aan.com
- **Consortium of Multiple Sclerosis Centers**—provides information on MS and clinical research. Also offers a registry for people with MS.
  www.mscare.org

Clinical Trials

- **National Institutes of Health**—provides information about clinical trials supported by the National Institutes of Health.
  www.nih.gov
  www.clinicaltrials.gov
- **CenterWatch Clinical Trials Listing Service**—provides information on clinical research and clinical trials; has separate sections for patients and healthcare professionals.
  www.centerwatch.com

Other Resources

- **Veterans Affairs MS Centers of Excellence**—established by the Department of Veterans Affairs, these centers are organized around clinical care, research and development, education and training, and information and telemedicine.
  www.va.gov/ms
- **Paralyzed Veterans of America**—source of information about the Americans with Disabilities Act, managed care, personal assistants, modifications, and more.
  www.pva.org

Pharmaceutical Companies

Pharmaceutical company Web pages are listed because they provide much useful information, but the viewer should be aware that these sites present information about the sponsor's drug product in a generally favorable light.

- **Avonex®**—information about the medication, provided by Biogen, Inc.
  www.avonex.com
- **MS ActiveSource** —information about MS, Avonex®, and patient assistance programs, provided by Biogen, Inc.
  www.msactivesource.com
- **Betaseron®**—information about the medication, provided by Berlex.
  www.betaseron.com
- **MS Pathways**—information about MS, Betaseron®, and patient assistance programs, provided by Berlex.
  www.mspathways.com
- **Copaxone®**—information about the medication, provided by Teva Neuroscience.
  www.mswatch.com
- **Shared Solutions**—information about MS, Copaxone®, and patient assistance programs, provided by Teva Neuroscience.
  www.sharesolutions.com
- **Rebif®**—information about the medication, provided by Serono, Inc.
  www.rebif.com
- **MSLifeLines**—information about MS, Rebif®, and patient assistance programs, provided by Serono, Inc.
  www.mslifelines.com
- **Novantrone®**—information about the medication, provided by Serono, Inc.
  www.novantrone.com
- **Medtronic, Inc.**—provides information about the Intrathecal Baclofen Pump for spasticity.
  www.medtronic.com

Recommended Books—
Newly Diagnosed Patients

- Bowling A: *Alternative Medicine and Multiple Sclerosis*. New York, Demos Medical Publishing, 2001.
  In an informative format, this book offers reliable information on the relevance, safety, and effectiveness of complementary and alternative therapies that are not typically considered in MS management, yet are widely used by individuals with MS.
- Holland NJ, Murray TJ, Reingold SC: *Multiple Sclerosis: A Guide for the Newly Diagnosed, 2nd Edition*. New York, Demos Medical Publishing, 2002.
  Written specifically for newly diagnosed people with MS, their families, and friends. Offers up-to-date information about living effectively with MS.
- Kalb RC: *Multiple Sclerosis: A Guide for Families*. New York: Demos Medical Publishing, 2000.
  This book demonstrates how families living with MS can create a balance between the needs of the members and those of the person with MS.
- Kalb RC: *Multiple Sclerosis: The Questions You Have, The Answers You Need, 2nd Edition*. New York, Demos Medical Publishing, 2000.
  Presented in a question-and-answer format, this book covers a broad spectrum of topics related to MS.
- Kraft GH, Catanzaro M: *Living With Multiple Sclerosis: A Wellness Approach, 2nd Edition*. New York, Demos Medical Publishing, 2000.
  This book provides information on such topics as symptom management, wellness management, emotional wellness, and social aspects.
- Schwartz SP: *300 Tips for Making Life with Multiple Sclerosis Easier*. New York, Demos Medical Publishing, 1999.
  This book is filled with suggestions, practical tips, and shortcuts the author learned from her own experiences.

Professional Books

- Halper J, Holland NJ: *Comprehensive Nursing Care in Multiple Sclerosis, 2nd Edition.* New York, Demos Medical Publishing, 2002.
  This definitive guide on the nursing care of people with MS provides an overview of the disease and its implications for nursing practice and examines specific arenas relating to nursing management.
- Polman CH, Thompson AJ, Murray TJ, et al: *Multiple Sclerosis: The Guide to Treatment and Management, 5th Edition.* New York, Demos Medical Publishing, 2001.
  This guide reviews the management of exacerbations, disease-modifying therapies, symptom management, and alternative therapies.
- Schapiro RT: *Managing the Symptoms of Multiple Sclerosis, 4th Edition.* New York, Demos Medical Publishing, 2003.
  This book explores the symptoms of MS and examines clinically tested and proven methods for the management of each.
- Holland NJ, Van den Noort S: *Multiple Sclerosis in Clinical Practice.* New York: Demos Medical Publishing, 1999.
  This book presents therapies that can be used by general neurologists and primary care physicians.

Index

NOTES

NOTES

NOTES

NOTES